# Feminism *Reconsidered*

*How Women are Exploited by Abortion*

*Gail M. Hamilton*

*Family of Man Publishing*
*Encino, California*

# Feminism Reconsidered
### How Women are Exploited by Abortion
### © 1994 by Gail M. Hamilton

All rights reserved.

First Edition
   Published by:

*Family of Man Publishing*
P. O. Box 17328
Encino, Ca., 91416-17328
818-718-1881

Printed and bound by KNI Incorporated, Anaheim, California.

Cover Design by Ed Elliott

Cataloging in Publication Data
Library of Congress 96-86068
ISBN number 0-9653315-7-1 (paper)
Index
Bibliography

Hamilton, Gail M.,
   An overview of feminism and legal abortion as it has affected American women and their families during the 1960's through the 1990's.

This book is dedicated to my friend, *Mary McCarty Stevens*, who was *joy and light,* and died much too soon.

**Her courage, calm, and insight were an inspiration to many.
Her dedication to the cause of life, in her own quiet way, was awesome.**

**May we meet again someday to whisper the names of Derrick and Olivia.**

# Feminism Reconsidered
## How Women are Exploited by Abortion

## Table of Contents

Preface-- i
Roe v. Wade-- 1
Planned Parenthood v. Casey-- 14
A World Upside Down-- 26
Abortion & the Politically-Correct-- 37
Abortion & the Medically-Correct-- 56
Used Women: Abortion & Big Business --74
Liberated Women-- 86
Looking for Daddy:Where in the World is Mom?-- 94
Sex Before Sixteen-- 107
The Media, Feminism and Abortion-- 123
Feminism and the Catholic Church-- 136
Dear Ms. Chairperson-- 147
Abortion & Religion-- 159
Toward a New Feminism-- 172
Epilogue-- 189
Update-- 196
Bibliography-- 201
Index-- 208

## Acknowledgments

I would like to acknowledge and thank my husband, Michael, who stands by me in the worst of times, and is always my friend.

And, I would like to thank my friends who encouraged me, and gave me some great ideas. Big Hugs: To Sandy Hlad, whose compassion is boundless. To Lorraine Mabbett, who "takes care" of me when I need someone to lean on. To Susan Farrell, who made me think I just might be able to write a book. And, to Pat Mullins, who never doubted.

## Preface

**"Life is a dynamic process. It welcomes anyone who takes up the invitation to be an active part of it. What we call the secret of happiness is no more a secret than our willingness to choose life..." Leo Buscaglia** [i]

Why should feminism be reconsidered? What has failed? Where has progress been made? How have feminist advances in the sexual revolution affected women, family life and our nation? Are we healthier, happier? Are we truly liberated, or have we been willingly deceived?

Women, at this point in time, should have all they want. Because of legal abortion, they can "control their own bodies." They have been empowered by those who champion their "reproductive rights." But, how many women have been irreparably damaged by one or more abortions? How many have been harmed by the lie that it is necessary to choose death for their unborn children, rather than choosing life? When did our values change?

In the 1960's, women began to seek sexual liberation. In the seventies, they were freed from "mandatory" childbirth by gaining legal access to abortion. In the eighties, their rights to abortion were even more firmly established. And, in 1992 this country elected a pro-abortion president, William Clinton.

Bill and Hillary Clinton have not disappointed those who think the way they do on the issues of abortion and feminism. This president's promotion of even more permissive abortions has been mind-boggling. So far, he has promoted federal funding of research on pre-born babies and "harvesting" of their tissue for transplantation. He attempted to reverse our country's policy against abortion-funding for military personnel and foreign countries. And, he successfully brought into the United States, RU-486 (the abortion pill) by the back door, through a research organization. All of Clinton's pro-abortion moves must warm the hearts of Planned Parenthood, the National Abortion Rights Action League, and the National Organization of Women, to name only a few.

To say that I was disappointed by the 1992 election is an understatement. *Devastated* is a more accurate word. I knew that with the Clintons in the White House, their influence in the press and Congress, would be very difficult to counteract. I found myself thinking that I needed to write a book concerning the truth about abortion. I didn't have much hope that anything so politically-incorrect would be published, but I did know that I needed to report what I have observed as a national tragedy.

Since 1970, I have spoken to thousands of women about their pregnancies and their abortion experiences. I began by helping to organize a chapter of the Right to Life League of Southern California. At first, we would speak to people we thought would be like-minded: those who might become active, sound the alarm, talk to others. We would go to pastors, schools, teachers, and friends, asking them to look at the pro-abortion atmosphere that was beginning to surround us. I would take my six-month-old daughter, Christine, with me as I sat in pastors' offices. I would squeeze in phone calls during her nap time.

Besides speaking about the issue when we could, some of us trained for a hotline that was designed to help women who were pregnant or thought they might be. We began to talk to women by phone at all hours of the day and night. A few years after that we opened a center, where we could counsel in person.

In 1984, I became the Director of the Pregnancy Counseling Center (now a clinic) in the San Fernando Valley. Our clinic is one of more than three thousand pregnancy centers in the United States. All of our services are free, and we try to help women and their unborn children in any way that we can. We are not well known to the general public. The liberal media doesn't acknowledge us because, if they did, they would have to give up the lie that we don't care about women. But, we are there, nevertheless, helping one woman at a time.

I have talked to hundreds of women seriously damaged from the physical and psychological effects of abortion. And, I have spoken to women whose lives were turned around because they made the decision to have their "unexpected" child—even though others had been pressuring them into the quick fix of an

# Preface

abortion. I found, over the years, that I would often speak with young women and teen girls about their self-respect and self-esteem. I would urge them to wait for sex until they were married. I would ask those who were pregnant to consider the fact that they would be very much alone with their abortion decision—for the rest of their lives.

I found out, unexpectedly, as I began to write this book, that I had become a feminist, though I probably wouldn't be accepted in any of the "better" feminist circles. I was surprised to discover, during my research, that Betty Friedan and I agreed on several women's issues, parting company, of course, on our abortion views. In her famous book, *The Feminine Mystique*,[ii] she advanced some very solid ideas for positive changes and equal rights for women. Her promotion of abortion, however, has been most unfortunate, and has polarized many who might have joined her campaign for women's rights.

I would like to propose a new type of feminism, one that claims equal rights, advantages, and respect for women, but admits men, children, and pre-born babies into the full circle of feminist causes.

There are, undeniably, basic differences between the sexes. A man is physically stronger than most women, and most women have the ability to conceive and bear children. I believe that God has designed the family structure, with the man as the head of the family, because of these differences. But, I also believe that the interpretation of what is meant by the term, "head of the family," has been skewed in order to deny women equality and respect. Many pregnant women I have counseled were more concerned about their boyfriend's or husband's life styles than they were concerned about themselves or their unborn children. How did they become women with so little self-esteem? Where did they get the idea that they were the only ones at fault; the only ones responsible for this unexpected pregnancy? Who told them that they had to "obey" this boyfriend or husband who wanted them to destroy their child? They learned to be submissive in their families, in their schools, and in their churches. The idea of the man being dominant, and having "ownership" privileges permeates many cultures.

Feminism, in our country, beginning in the last century, was headed in the right direction, but took the wrong path when feminists began to seek empowerment, rather than equality. Many told women that they no longer needed marriage, that they have the right to be as "sexually free" as men have always been. When teen girls and women, encouraged by a liberal society, believe they will find freedom with several different sexual partners; and when they are told that they have the right to destroy any unborn children conceived from even the most casual relationships, they are deceived. They are the losers. Men are still the winners.

Modern feminism, as promoted in the last three decades, has failed <u>precisely because of this sexual revolution</u> and its attendant, easy, legal access to abortion. Rather than "emancipating" women, it has entangled and enslaved them so completely that the truth is not even seen by women who have been damaged by their abortion experiences. Some women are still telling their sisters that abortion and a free sexual lifestyle are liberating!

Women have been led down the proverbial garden path by their feminist sisters. What they have found, however, when they were looking for the freedom of an open meadow, is a thick forest of lies, abandonment, and loneliness.

I firmly believe that a path leading toward true equality still needs to be there, but that it must make a sharp turn. I would like to propose a new feminism that can begin right now. I am willing to stand as politically-incorrect today, in the hope that men and women will listen to the truth about abortion and its harmful effects, while still pursuing equality for all women. My hope is that with this knowledge, that new path will be taken, one that leads to a more positive future for the family of man, of which we are all a part. My hope is for a world where we choose life, even in the most difficult of circumstances.

---

[i] Leo Buscaglia,, *Bus 9 to Paradise*, Fawcett-Columbine, NY, 1986, p. 154.
[ii] Betty Friedan, *The Feminine Mystique*, 20th Anniversary edition, W. W. Norton & Co., NY, 1983.

# *Roe v. Wade*

**Once there was an Archer
And there was a minute
When He shot a shaft
On a New Departure.
Then He must have laughed:
Comedy was in it.
For the Game He hunted
Was the non-existence,
And His shaft got blunted
On its non-resistance.**
       ____ Robert Frost[1]

Roe v . Wade,[2] the Supreme Court decision handed down on January 22, 1973, ruled that there is a constitutional right of privacy that includes women's rights to abortion. Harry Blackmun, et al, by the stroke of a pen, transformed the crime of abortion into a constitutional right! He and his fellow justices in the majority opinion spoke of a *penumbra* that emanated from the right to privacy found in our Constitution.

In Katz v. United States, a 1967 case cited in support of its decision in Roe, the court noted in a footnote that: *"Virtually every governmental action interferes with personal privacy to some degree. The question in each case is whether that interference violates a command of the U. S. Constitution."*[3]

The Supreme justices could not find anything in the Constitution that protects human life at conception or throughout the nine months of gestational development. They found that laws against abortion violated individual privacy--and that included the privacy to take the life of one's own child, in utero. But, what about our unborn citizens? Aren't they persons? Aren't they alive?

The Court's answer was that they couldn't define either personhood or viability exactly, so they gave the full benefit of the doubt to women and their doctors. The unborn child, who might be a person *or* viable, (according to the justices' non-definition) can't defend himself in either case, simply because of his environment and stage of development.

Whether or not a privacy right that includes the right to

abortion actually exists in our Constitution became a moot point because the majority opinion found *emanations from a penumbra.* The Justices who voted with Harry Blackmun in the majority opinion were Potter Steward, William Brennan, Lewis Powell, William Douglas, Warren Burger, and Thurgood Marshall. The Justices who dissented were William Rehnquist and Byron White.

Never before has the fabric of a society been so weakened and torn by a "penumbra." This decision, fashioned out of whole cloth continues to sanction the killing of over one and a half million children per year! The archer's shaft has certainly been blunted on the non-existence. But there isn't any comedy in it--only tragedy.

When moral good is fashioned from social expediency and political cost-effectiveness, no one is safe--not the aged, infirm, handicapped, or pre-born children. This penumbra has cost our country thirty-six million lives, so far, and has cost (at least) that many women their peace of mind. It has also set the stage for euthanasia, assisted suicide, fetal research and harvesting of pre-born organs for transplant, and a general disregard for human beings at any point in their existence.

I recently found, in some well-buried correspondence, a letter I had written to Norman Cousins on October 19, 1971, one year and a few months before Roe v. Wade. Mr. Cousins was, at that time, the Editor of *The Saturday Review*, and had written an article about a prison riot that had occurred in Attica, New York. The treatment and gunning down of prisoners there had been decried generally by the press for its disregard of human life. I was especially encouraged by a paragraph Mr. Cousins had written in his article that called for respect for all individuals. He was especially concerned about the government's treatment of all of its citizens.

*"No idea or principle is more basic to that government than that the value of a man's life transcends his pedigree or pigmentation or politics or personality or property. Nor is any notion more alien in such a society than that some men have the right to kick other men around because their power to do so is sanctioned by qualitative standards."*[4]

What a beautiful defense of all life, including unborn life! Or, so I thought. I wrote Mr. Cousins and told him that I agreed with him wholeheartedly and passionately, and that I hoped that he would be open to writing an article in defense of the unborn using his profoundly-stated ideas. This was fifteen months before Roe v. Wade, but the media had already started arguing the case for abortion long before this particular article was written. I was hoping that his would be a well-respected voice in the other direction.

I was, of course, disappointed. After the eloquence of his article about the treatment of prisoners and their rights, I expected more. His personal letter to me included rhetoric that could have been the standard for all the form letters I have since received from pro-abortion "thinkers."

In his letter, dated October 26, 1971, he said,

*"The choice is not, I fear, between abortion and no abortion. The choice is, to put it bluntly, between legalized abortions, and illegal abortions on kitchen tables in the back woods--abortions that are only too likely to kill both mother and unborn infant."*[5]

How disappointng. Why was he equivocating? We each wrote one more letter, neither of us getting too far in our arguments.

Mr. Cousins later wrote a book, *Anatomy of an Illness As Perceived by the Patient*,[6] about a serious virus that he contracted and how he dealt with (and overcame) the physical and emotional devastation of ankylosing spondylitis. The connective tissue in his spine was deteriorating, but he decided to fight this disease in an unconventional manner. Mr. Cousins seemed to be an interesting man, one I would have liked to meet. I never did, but I often wonder if he changed his mind about that letter he had written so many years earlier. Possibly, his brush with an early death changed his point of view on the value of life for all, including the unborn. I sincerely hope so.

His "kitchen-table" argument is still used as the *raison d'être* for continued abortion on demand, for any reason. The same debate is used as a graphic example to demonstrate that anyone who is against *safe*, *legal* abortion doesn't care about women or the risks to their life and health. Nothing could be farther from the truth. Everyone who would like this nation to return to sanity by rejecting abortion as a legal right cares very much for women and their children!

The ugly placards and ads promoting safe abortions that depict an unconscious woman and a bloody hanger are half-true, however. Just replace the hanger with a scissors, forceps, cannula and a suction respirator machine and you have the truth about legal abortion. Just the year before Roe v. Wade, thirty-nine "official" deaths were reported from illegal abortions. Now that one and a half million abortions take place yearly, how many deaths and maimings do you think there are? How many are "officially" reported?

One of the great lies promoted by abortion activists is that abortion is safer than childbirth. Not considering the ultimate complication of death, the medical risks inherent in abortion are far more dangerous than those of pregnancy for healthy women. Infection, perforated uterus, pelvic inflammatory disease, hemorrhage, and a dramatically increased risk of future miscarriages are among the most frequent side effects. A common occurrence is incomplete abortion, which, if not corrected very soon after the initial procedure with a second abortion, can lead to serious infection.

Roe v. Wade, promoted by feminists and their feminist agenda, was supposed to be so liberating for women. They have, instead, become enslaved by the perceived sexual freedom that they were granted by this judicial activism. Who actually wins? Who is liberated by an abortion? The father of the aborted child walks away--free of responsibility, free of any commitment to the woman or his child. She is abandoned and alone. Very few relationships survive the abortion experience. Often, a teen girl's parents are saved the embarrassment of an unwed daughter having a child. Their social standing is preserved at the country club. And, of course, the abortion doctor makes out, (like a bandit) several times a day--making a *healthy* living by assembly-line abortions. Everybody is free and clear, except the woman who has to live with physical and emotional damage, and the memories of a traumatic, violent experience that will do everything but solve her problems.

The justices went so far in their determination of a constitutional right to abortion that they included in their ruling a very specific trimester schedule. I don't know why they bothered as abortion is actually legal throughout nine months of a pregnancy.

In the first trimester, there can be no interference by law. A woman and her doctor need only have the desire for an abortion and the means to do it. In the second trimester, the State can only regulate against the abortion procedure in consideration of the health of the mother. In other words, if there were a risk to the woman's health, there could be a legal indication that the procedure should not be performed. This is the reason that most abortion mills, the 10-minute varieties, farm out the later abortions. They don't want the responsibility for care of a woman who wants a mid- or late-term abortion.

The State *may* protect the life of the fetus in the third trimester, but it does not necessarily have to because the "health" (psychological, most often) of the mother supersedes the right to life of the unborn seventh, eighth or nine-month child, even when his humanness (because he looks like a baby) cannot be denied., but the weight of "possible" viability was not used to offer even a little protection for the unborn child. I heard President Reagan use the following example once: If a person were hit by a car and was lying unconscious or dead in the street, the benefit of the doubt would certainly be given to him. He would be presumed alive for awhile, at least. Certainly, we, as onlookers or paramedics would attempt to save his life. He asked why this wasn't true for the unborn child. Not so with Roe v. Wade. The exact moment of viability cannot be determined, according to the supreme justices. Therefore, all consideration is given to the woman and her doctor, none to the unborn child.

Roe v. Wade stated that individual State legislatures could not prohibit post-viability abortions if the health of the mother were a concern. Doe v. Bolton,[7] the companion case, defined health so that it would include emotional, familial, and psychological well-being. This locked in the right to abortion through all nine months of pregnancy. In other words, a nervous woman's personality is sufficient indication for her right to a late-term abortion. Or, the loss of a woman's comfortable lifestyle might affect her well-being, and therefore she is legally able to obtain an abortion.

How an individual's privacy (to kill her unborn child) ever became the overriding interest when another person's right to life is totally ignored, still baffles me. A fetus (from the Latin for young one) is not a person? At eighteen days after conception the unborn child's heart starts beating. At forty days, brain waves can be detected. From this time on, the child only develops and refines. Nothing new will be added. If this girl or boy is not a living human being, and, thus, a person, what is it?

Personhood comes with the territory of our humanness. It is part of the whole. To say that personhood arrives only at an arbitrary point in time determined by a Supreme Court, a doctor, or a pregnant woman is absurd. We all come with personhood. To be conceived by two human beings and then to develop as a human being during the pregnancy, makes us human. Personhood is an intrinsic part of our humanity. We were not animals in our pre-born state and then at a certain point in time metamorphosed into humans. Each of us, born or pre-born, is unique. Each of us, intrinsically, is a person.

The personhood of the unborn child has become increasingly visible with the advent of ultrasound imaging, giving us moving pictures of the pre-born baby and its life inside the womb. He moves, sucks, his heart can be seen beating. Each in-utero child is different in its limited actions. It not only has personhood, but it already has personality.

In 1989, in Webster v. Reproductive Health Services,[8] the Court allowed some restrictions to abortion in Missouri. Upheld was the law against public facilities or employees participating in abortion and a law requiring a test for viability of the unborn after twenty weeks. The Supreme Court let stand the preamble in Missouri's law that states **life begins at conception**. There is some hope for other states to follow similar legislation eventually.

The right of privacy, and thus the right to abortion, in California is so well-established that even if Roe v. Wade were overturned, our State Constitution would still guarantee legal abortions. In 1967, the Therapeutic Abortion Act was signed by Governor Ronald Reagan. Then, in 1972, a privacy provision was added, by vote, to our State constitution. There had been nowhere in the ballot arguments for this constitutional amendment any hint of the pervasiveness or the convoluted reasoning that would be used by these two pieces of legislation to entrench legal abortion into our State government. There was nowhere any indication in the California constitutional privacy provision, as advertised, that it was anything more than a protection of our rights from the intrusiveness of government and business, and their incessant information-gathering. Simply by changing *men* to *people* and adding the word *privacy*, abortion rights were established by this amendment in *Article 1, Section 1 of the Constitution of the State of California*.

In 1981, in Committee to Defend Reproductive Rights v. Myers,[9] the California Supreme Court interpreted the right to privacy to mean the right to kill an unborn child by legal abortion. This decision also mandated that funds must be available for abortions through Medi-Cal (California's State-funded health insurance), so long as funds were being used for pre-natal and childbirth services, as well.

Why should a woman have this breathtaking power over another human being, her unborn child? Why should she be supported and applauded for her decision not to bring her child into an imperfect world (a phrase I have heard time and again as an excuse for abortion)? And, if she should have this power, why should another person, a drive-by shooter or an armed robber, for example, be prosecuted for murder in the death of an unborn child? Because the mother, perhaps, wanted the child? Or should the shooter or robber be prosecuted because he is not a doctor, performing an abortion? What if he were a doctor?

Say, for example, a doctor and his wife were having marital problems and he decided to abort his unborn child against his wife's wishes. And, if he succeeds? What would be his crime? He is a doctor and the father of the unborn. Why should he be prosecuted for anything? Rape, possibly? Shouldn't he have the right to kill his unborn child? His wife does.

Of course, then we come to the "*It isn't human until it's viable*" argument. Why isn't it? As noted above, eighteen days after conception a heartbeat can be detected. At this point in time, a woman isn't even sure she's pregnant. A woman with an irregular menstrual cycle probably hasn't even thought about being late. Again, at forty days, brain waves can be detected. This isn't even six weeks into the pregnancy, the gestational point required for safe abortions!

If the fetus isn't human, what is it? If it isn't living and growing, why abort it? If viability is based on whether or not a child can breathe, take nourishment, process it, and develop and grow on her own, then abortions should be legal for about two and a half years after birth. Why, if the circumstances warranted it, such as the health of her mother, couldn't a one-year-old child be aborted? A toddler is not able to provide for her own sustenance and health.

If her mother were not able to care for her, society would find another caretaker, nourishment provider, and hopefully a loving substitute for her in adoption or legal guardianship. Why can't that be true as an alternative to abortion? The lists of potential adoptive parents is astoundingly and agonizingly long.

Why should a child be denied his life because his mother doesn't want him? Or, because she is afraid that if she carries him within her body for nine months it might be painful to part with her baby once she sees him? She thinks that by ending his life before a time when she might *miss* him, before she sees him, she will be spared the pain of the loss of her child. How very mistaken she is!

The Roe of Roe v. Wade was Norma McCorvey, of Texas. She, at first, claimed that she was raped and impregnated as a result of rape. She later revealed that that was untrue. Luckily for her daughter, Roe v. Wade was too late. Norma gave birth to a girl, who was given to adoptive parents.

I have seen Norma McCorvey for brief moments over the years on television. She has been presented as a useful tool by activists on various politically-correct occasions. She has been packaged and put on a convenient shelf, to be taken down when needed. She seems to be someone who, at the very least, is inarticulate, or someone with a low IQ. Sometimes during her public appearances she appears sleepy, unsure of what is happening. She has been used by those who claim to be her champions. I feel sorry for her.

When the Supreme Court of the United States found a privacy reason for abortion hidden somewhere in the folds of the Constitution they declared open season on thirty-six million, so far, of our tiniest, weakest citizens. Never mind that the Bill of Rights states that all men have an inalienable right to life. What rights should a blob of tissue have (albeit, a blob whose heart has already been beating for six weeks or longer)? The justices said, in effect, that a woman's privacy or lifestyle should take precedence over another person's life.

Now, if there is such little regard for human beings at this stage, how much respect will there be for the older person who no longer is a productive contributor to society, but, in fact, may be very inconvenient to his or her family or to the state? It may soon be common for physicians to perform euthanasia or assist in suicides. It isn't difficult to see how easy it will be to get rid of someone who is no longer productive, or who has never been productive. What about a handicapped person? Why not offer "death with dignity" to someone who is only a strain on our emotional lives and our pocketbooks?

Abortion has become fashionable. Indeed, a whole generation of our young people have grown up thinking that abortion is a moral good, there for their convenience, a popular remedy for "playing around." Another, new moral good has been introduced into our society, an atrocity of such dimensions it's difficult to comprehend unless you actually see and hear the descriptions of it. It's known as the D and X (dilation and extraction) procedure, or a partial-birth abortion. Unborn children are kept alive long enough to be used for laboratory experiments or for harvesting of their usable organs.

The following is a series of sketches that details Martin Haskell's method, which he "perfected" for late term abortions and for harvesting organs from the unborn.[10]

10                              Feminism Reconsidered

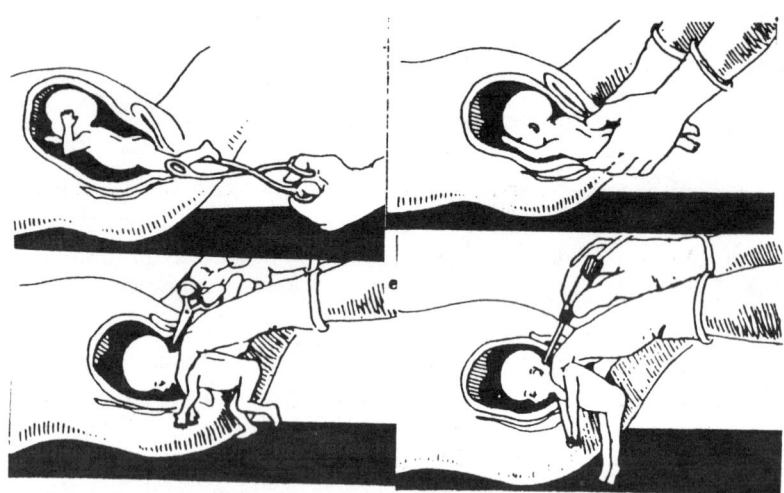

The abortionist jams scissors into the baby's skull. The scissors are then opened to enlarge the hole.

The scissors are removed and a suction cathether is inserted. The child's brains are sucked out. The baby is then "evacuated."

Used with permission, Life Advocate Magazine, Oregon

After three days of dilating the patient's cervix by means of Dilapan dilators, the fetus is scanned by ultrasound probe in order to locate the lower extremities. Haskell uses large forceps to grasp a leg and pull it into the vagina. He uses his fingers to deliver the other leg. He can then experiment or harvest organs while the child is still alive, but still, *technically*, in the process of being aborted. When he's ready to finish the abortion, he locates the skull and forces a curved scissors into the base of the child's neck. The scissors are opened to enlarge the hole. He removes the scissors and inserts a suction catheter to suck out the baby's brains. With the skull emptied, the baby is then removed completely.

Haskell developed this technique for killing unborn babies as old as six months and weighing as much as two pounds. The method was introduced by him in a paper given at the National Abortion Federation Risk Management Seminar on September 13, 1992 in Dallas. His technique is designed to keep the babies alive for as long as possible by keeping them attached by the umbilical cord to the placenta, technically still in the process of an abortion. But, in reality, using an unborn child for utilitarian purposes before killing it.

Though some try to paint this gruesome abortion as a necessary one to save the lives of mothers, in the Analysis portion of Haskell's paper, he mentions that this procedure is good because only local anesthetic is needed and the appointment scheduling is convenient!

Just imagine being the mother of that child during the abortion. While you are lying on the surgical table, your child dangles, feet-first, out of your vagina while his brains or other organs are being removed for experimentation or transplantation. What are you feeling? Will the humanitarian purposes of your "useful" fetus neutralize in your subconscious the reality of the abortion, the death of your child? For how long?

That terrible decision on January 22, 1973, by a few men, has changed the course of this nation. Not only was violence legalized and condoned, it was embraced. And, more often than not, women are its victims. Those who champion legal abortion as good for women are mistaken, at the very least. Or they are disingenuous and have a hidden agenda for promoting abortion. Abortion certainly has become big business. The doctor can make a really fast buck off of the same woman (many times). The abortionist is the only winner! The losers are the unborn child, who has no chance at life and his mother who will be damaged either emotionally, physically, or both. Women are not empowered or freed by abortion--they are enslaved and duped.

When I see young girls or women who are facing a possible problem pregnancy, I want to hug each one and talk to them as a mother might when discussing important decisions. I want to say, "Honey, take time to think a minute before entering into a sexual relationship without marriage. If he tells you to trust him--don't! Because, even if he sincerely means what he's saying at the moment, that little piece of paper called a marriage license that is so ridiculed by young people today, *is* a true test of trust and commitment. And without it, he can walk when things get difficult. If you get pregnant, most of the time you are left with the responsibility, the pain, and the ultimate decision of life or death by yourself. Everybody "walks" but you. Think about it. Not having sex with him doesn't mean you love him any less, it simply means you care about both of you and a long-term relationship built on love and respect, not on sex alone." Corny, they might say to me--it doesn't apply to today's young people. That's too bad, I would say to them, because it's still the truth.

Roe v. Wade was a grave error, a mistake that has cost the lives of millions of unborn human beings, and has caused the loss of emotional and physical well-being for millions of women, as well. If we ever return to sanity, we will see a new day dawn in a government and a people that respects and protects all human life. If we don't, things will only worsen and become more violent, more dangerous, where our streets, our hospitals, even our homes will not offer safety for any of us. In a prophetic book in 1972, *Abortion and Social Justice*,[11] Thomas Hilgers talked about the consequences of abortion on demand for this country.

*"The position that our law takes on abortion indicates the position it will take on euthanasia, genetic engineering, cloning, and all of the difficult human life problems facing our society in the years ahead. Those who argue for the unborn child's right to life are arguing not only for the unborn child, but for the civil right to life of every human being--the mentally ill, the aged, the genetically incompetent, the idle, the useless. If the law abandons the protection of the civil rights of the innocent child in the womb, it will one day abandon its protection of the civil right to life of the mentally incompetent, the senile and the hopelessly ill. It will abandon its protection of your civil rights."*[12]

[1] Robert Frost, "Version," from *In the Clearing*, Holt, Rinehart and Winston, 1965, p. 37.
[2] Roe v. Wade, 410 U. S. 113, 1973.
[3] Katz v. United States, 389 U.S. 347,350 S. Ct.507 (1967).
[4] Norman Cousins, in *The Saturday Review*, Oct. 16, 1971.
[5] Norman Cousins, from a personal letter to the author.
[6] Norman Cousins, *Anatomy of an Illness As Perceived by the Patient*, W. W. Norton & Company, Inc., New York, N.Y.., 173 pp.
[7] Doe v. Bolton, 410 U.S., 179 [1973].
[8] Webster, Attorney General of Missouri v. Reproductive Health Services, et al., Court of Appeals, 8th Circuit, 88-605, [1989].
[9] Committee to Defend Reproductive Rights v. Myers, 29 CAL. 3D 252 [1981].
[10] Reprinted from the Right to Life Educational Foundation, Inc. Bulletin, March, 1993, published by the Cincinnati Right to Life, Cincinnati, Ohio.
[11] Thomas W. Hilgers, in Hilgers and Horan, *Abortion & Social Justice*, Sheed & Ward, Inc., 1972.
[12] Ibid., p. 106.

# *Planned Parenthood v. Casey*

"Abortion and totalitarianism both represent new possibilities of some men's power over others, and both are defended by certain ideologies of 'progress.' We hear of human 'autonomy' and of man's 'control of his own destiny.' But the autonomy is enjoyed by a select (or self-selected) few, and the control is exercised by a shrinking elite; those who are powerless, whether unborn children or the subjects of a totalist dictatorship, simply don't count."[1]_____Joseph Sobran

When legislation that offered some protection to the unborn child, and somewhat restricted a woman's abortion rights, was passed in Pennsylvania, Planned Parenthood decided to take action against the State and the Governor, Robert P. Casey. The appeal eventually reached the Supreme Court. The Court handed down its decision in the case of Planned Parenthood of Southeastern Pennsylvania, et al v. Robert P. Casey, Governor of Pennsylvania, et al,[2] in July of 1992.

The following paragraph is an excerpt from Justices O'Connor, Kennedy, and Souter's opinion. I find it one of the most revealing, most offensive, and most frightening of all the pro-abortion rhetoric I have ever read. The idea that utilitarianism should be a bottom-line for the continuation of the wholesale slaughter of the next generation is unconscionable.

*"The Roe rule's limitation on state power could not be repudiated without serious inequity to people who, for two decades of economic and social developments, <u>have organized intimate relationships and made choices that define their places in society, in reliance on the availability of abortion in the event that contraception should fail.</u> The ability of women to participate equally in the economic and social life of the Nation has been facilitated by their ability to control their reproductive lives. The Constitution serves human values, and while the effect of reliance on Roe cannot be exactly measured, neither can the certain costs of overruling Roe for people who have ordered their thinking and living around that case be dismissed."* (emphasis added) [3]

Do we really understand from the foregoing paragraph that people have "ordered their thinking and living" around the fact that abortion (the direct killing of their unborn children) is a

# Planned Parenthood v. Casey

back-up for their failed contraceptive practices? And, because people have depended on the ability to do this legally for so long that it would be very difficult for them to no longer have the legal right to abortion? Do I understand from this convoluted reasoning that not having that right might inconvenience them?

Especially interesting is the phrase, "...in the event that contraception should fail..." Does this mean if a couple had not been using contraception, they would not be eligible for an abortion? What about all of the hundreds of thousands of men and women who don't use contraception regularly because it's inconvenient or uncomfortable, or because they are only 14 years old and "it" can't happen to them? Do the justices really believe that the only women having abortions are upscale, yuppie, career women who might lose their promotion at the office if they are pregnant? Do they think that every fertile female in America walks around in an always-readied state of contraception?

In the case of Planned Parenthood of Southeastern Pennsylvania v. Casey, Justice Blackmun, the chief author of Roe v. Wade, restated his original findings in that case to support his rejection of the Pennsylvania law that was more protective of the unborn child. If Blackmun ever changed his mind and found that children in the womb have a right to even minimal legal protection, he would probably not publicly say so. Why not? Because of his intellectual pride. This man is egotistically "stuck" with his deadly decision.

In a revealing closing statement in the Casey decision, Blackmun is very obvious: he sees his role clearly and boastfully, in past and future history. He states:

> "In one sense, the Court's approach is worlds apart from that of the Chief Justice and Justice Scalia. And yet, in another sense, the distance between the two approaches is short--the distance is but a single vote.
> "I am 83 years old. I cannot remain on this Court forever, and when I do step down, the confirmation process for my successor well may focus on the issue before us today. That, I regret, may be exactly where the choice between the two worlds will be made."[4]

Further evidence of subjective, pro-active thinking and judgment is seen in the following statement:

> "State restrictions on abortion violate a woman's right of privacy in two ways. First, compelled continuation of a pregnancy infringes upon a woman's right to bodily integrity by imposing substantial physical intrusions and significant risks of physical harm. During pregnancy, women experience dramatic physical changes and a wide range of health consequences. Labor and delivery pose additional health risks and physical demands..."[5]

I don't exactly find this shocking--laughable would be the better term. Ever since humans arrived on this planet, the normal, natural manner of procreation and the results thereof have been the process of growth and development of the unborn child inside of his mother. There he is nourished and sustained as he develops. The fact that pregnancy and birth are presented as an illness, an intrusion, a handicap, an unnatural, risky sequence of events, must be a joke. He's got to be kidding. Or is this his compassionate side?

The next section defines some of the "real" restrictions that might hamper a woman and her lifestyle, her plans, her happiness.

> "Further, when the State restricts a woman's right to terminate her pregnancy, it deprives a woman of the right to make her own decision about reproduction and family planning--critical life choices that this Court long has deemed central to the right of privacy. The decision to terminate or continue a pregnancy has no less an impact on a woman's life than decisions about contraception or marriage, 410, U.S., at 153. Because motherhood has a dramatic impact on a woman's educational prospects, employment opportunities, and self-determination, restrictive abortion laws deprive her of basic control over her life."[6]

> "...State restrictions on abortion compel women to continue pregnancies they otherwise might terminate. By restricting the right to terminate pregnancies, the State <u>conscripts women's bodies</u> into its service, forcing women to continue their pregnancies, suffer the pains of childbirth, and in most instances, provide years of maternal care. The State does not compensate women for their services; instead, it assumes that they owe this duty as a matter of course. This assumption--that women can simply be forced to accept the 'natural' status and incidents of motherhood--appears to rest upon a conception of women's role that has triggered the protection of the Equal Protection Clause. See e.g., Mississippi Univ. for Women v. Hogan, 158 U.S. 718,724-726 (1982); Craig v. Boren 429 U. S. 190, 198-199 (1976). The joint opinion recognizes that these assumptions about women's place in society 'are no longer consistent with our understanding of the family, the individual, or

*the Constitution.' Ante, at 55."* [7]

    I think Blackmun was appallingly clear and so *politically-correct* in his intentions with these two paragraphs. He didn't even attempt to disguise his feminist language. He states that if the government were to limit abortion, it would be restricting a woman's *right to privacy* because it would restrict her decisions about reproduction and family planning. However, what he totally ignores is the fact that she has already reproduced. She chose to do so. If her method of family planning failed, whether through human or mechanical error, the fact still remains that she is pregnant, has reproduced, and what is living within her is another human being, her child. No one is guaranteed perfect results in life's circumstances. Money-back deals might come with things you buy through the mail or at J. C. Penney's, but life doesn't guarantee perfection. Indeed, it guarantees difficulties and imperfections.

    He says that, "because a woman might be restricted in her educational or employment opportunities, she should not be denied the right to an abortion." Think about it. Is anyone really denied the right to education or employment when she is pregnant? Most women do not live in a vacuum. They can work and go to school, even if it's easier without the pregnancy. Pregnancy is not a disease or a handicap. Neither is motherhood.

    He thinks that *forced* childbirth conscripts women's bodies into service. First of all, she was not forced (unless she was raped) into sexual intercourse. She chose that freely. Her becoming a mother is a natural result of intercourse if she is fertile, and if the intercourse occurred during that time of her menstrual cycle.

    *Enslavement* and *conscription* are very strange terms to use about pregnancy and motherhood. One's absolute power over another, enslavement, could not be more fully illustrated than in the right to take another person's life, as sanctioned by the State. Abortion may be found in his penumbra of the emanating right to privacy, but what about the unborn child's right to privacy? Shouldn't his very first environment be protected? We have environmentalists whose goal is to protect our natural resources and animal life? Shouldn't a child's life be more valuable and, therefore, protected by the State, too?

The most perfect answer to these ridiculous statements by Blackmun is found in the minority opinion of Rehnquist, Scalia, White, and Thomas as follows:

> *"The joint opinion thus turns to what can only be described as an unconventional--and unconvincing--notion of reliance, a view based on the surmise that the availability of abortion since Roe has led to 'two decades of economic and social developments' that would be undercut if the error of Roe were recognized. Ibid. The joint opinion's assertion of this fact is undeveloped and totally conclusory. In fact, one can not be sure to what economic and social developments the opinion is referring. Surely it is dubious to suggest that women have reached their 'places in society' in reliance upon Roe, rather than as a result of their determination to obtain higher education and compete with men in the job market, and of society's increasing recognition of their ability to fill positions that were previously thought to be reserved only for men."*[8]

The belief that women have achieved equality by determination and talent is far more supportive of women as individuals (**more feminist**) than Blackmun's notion of women who were freed from "slavery" by abortion, and, thus, are able to climb the corporate ladder.

Planned Parenthood, in its defense of bringing suit against the Governor of Pennsylvania, offers the following statements about the law in that state that required a 24-hour waiting period for abortions.

> *"Many Americans believe that pregnant women should have time to carefully consider whether to have an abortion. Under the guise of furthering this goal, some states have enacted legislation requiring women to wait a prescribed amount of time--generally 24 or 48 hours--after they have given informed consent, before the abortion actually can be performed. Rather than aiding women, waiting periods have been shown to increase the health risk of the abortion, create logistical problems, and increase the cost of the procedure."*[9]

In the same fact sheet, Planned Parenthood tells us how women do, in fact, carefully consider their abortion decision.

> *"Women having abortions carefully consider their decisions in light of their individual circumstances and whether they are ready to*

have children..."[10]

Nothing could be farther from the truth. Often, women have come to our clinic for an abortion appointment. They had made a date and time to abort, but weren't even sure of the name of the facility where they were going to do it. How much serious thought was given to this "procedure?"

They were emotional, upset and certainly not in a frame of mind to make any important decisions about their future or the future of their unborn children. To ask a woman to wait for one day to consider whether or not to have an abortion is not an undue burden. It's only good medical practice.

Often, when a woman wants to find out if she is pregnant with a crisis pregnancy and whether or not she wants to keep it, she will call Planned Parenthood or an abortion clinic for a pregnancy test. They "sensitively" ask if she will be terminating with them. Their first question is not when was the first day of her last period, but, "Will you be terminating with us?" --as if it were a given, as if they don't want to be bothered if she is not!

A woman came to us several years ago who had gone to a Planned Parenthood Clinic, trying to get some information on their abortion procedure. She was in the waiting room, trying to talk to an assistant behind the glass window. The clinic worker was reluctant to give her information about the abortion, relating to methods, anesthesia, and recovery. She finally said that if the woman would bring in her $350.00 cash, she would be given that information. So much for careful consideration! You need to commit to the abortion before you can find out about it.

Some of the difficulties cited for women having to wait were presented in this information sheet:

*"The logistics of arranging a second appointment may be cumbersome or even prohibitive for many of the 68 percent of patients who are working (and would have to arrange additional time off from work), the 42 percent who already have children (and would have to make child care arrangements), and the 31 percent who are in school. On average, students miss an additional two days of classes in order to return for a second visit."*[11]

We are talking about traumatic surgery here, not about a

trip to the orthodontist. If the decision whether or not to take your unborn child's life can't take more than twenty-four hours because it might be an inconvenience, well, that's too bad!

Blackmun, in Planned Parenthood v. Casey, writes about women's place in society, and offers that the assumptions of natural status and incidents of motherhood are no longer consistent with our understanding of the family, the individual, or the Constitution. In other words, if the *our* he refers to is the government, then they have reconsidered natural things and have decided *against* nature. If the *our* refers only to himself, then he needs to take a marriage and family course at the local community college. If he means to affect society by changing the natural, social structure of the family, then his decision is not based on law, but on his own pro-active, social-engineering agenda.

In Planned Parenthood v. Casey, the opinions of Chief Justice Rehnquist and Justices Scalia, Thomas, and White demonstrate the very essence of the difference between the right of privacy when no other individual's rights are involved and the hypothetical right of privacy that includes abortion.

*"In Roe v. Wade, the Court recognized a 'guarantee of personal privacy' which 'is broad enough to encompass a woman's decision whether or not to terminate her pregnancy.' 410 U.S., at 152-153. We are now of the view that, in terming this right fundamental, the Court in Roe read the earlier opinions upon which it based its decision much too broadly. Unlike marriage, procreation and contraception, abortion 'involves the purposeful termination of potential life.' Harris v. McRae, 448 U. S. 297, 325 (1980). The abortion decision must therefore 'be recognized as sui generis, different in kind from the others that the Court has protected under the rubric of personal or family privacy and autonomy.' Thornburgh v. American College of Obstetricians and Gynecologists, supra, at 792 (White, J., dissenting). One cannot ignore the fact that a woman is not isolated in her pregnancy, and that the decision to abort necessarily involves the destruction of a fetus. See Michael H. v. Gerald D., supra, at 124, n. 4 (To look "at the act which is assertedly the subject of a liberty interest in isolation from its effect upon other people [is] like inquiring whether there is a liberty interest in firing a gun where the case at hand happens to involve its discharge into another person's body')."*[12]

Here lies the fundamental argument against abortion on demand: there is no consideration of the rights of the human being, who just happens to be *in utero*. Abortion is not a victimless crime. The other person involved, the unborn child, is most vulnerable and in need of the protection of the State. To say that a woman is pregnant with something other than a human being is ludicrous.

What if a man were to break into a dog kennel and kill three pregnant prize bitches? If he were caught, would he be prosecuted and ordered to make compensation for three dogs, or would the law compel him to compensate the kennel owner for, say, eighteen in-utero puppies,--potential champions and potential revenue? Probably, at the very least, $12,000 (or more) would be demanded. Are dogs more valuable than humans, more worthy of legal safeguards? I guess so.

Should one be uncomfortable with the comparison of unborn dogs and unborn humans? I don't like it much, but it illustrates our puzzling value system. The law, as it stands now, protects unborn animals because they are wanted and useful. In California, we spend an inordinate amount of money, time, and energy on California condor eggs, trying to preserve the species. In one lab, scientists are carefully nurturing a bird egg that has only a small chance of survival, while in another they are harvesting human baby parts by means of "careful abortion" with the final result being the death of the unborn human. To say that we have our values upside down is an understatement, at the very least!

The extent of the value one human being holds for another should not determine whether or not the *other* (the unborn) is wanted. Many old people are a burden and unwanted. And, I assure you that they are next on the list of burdensome individuals. Just witness how narrowly the euthanasia bill, Proposition 161, was defeated in California in November of 1992. Let's face it, we are all affected by disregard for human life.

From the minority opinion in Planned Parenthood v. Casey, the argument against legal precedent, a caution against finding specific entitlements in a document, (the Constitution), that were not there, and the reiteration of the fact that the Supreme Court is there to decide and interpret the Constitution in general terms is embodied in a few succinct paragraphs written by Chief

Justice Rehnquist, Justices White, Scalia, and Thomas:

*"...By the turn of the century virtually every State had a law prohibiting or restricting abortion on its books. By the middle of the present century, a liberalization trend had set in. But 21 of the restrictive abortion laws in effect in 1868 were still in effect in 1973 when Roe was decided, and an overwhelming majority of the States prohibited abortion unless necessary to preserve the life or health of the mother. Roe v. Wade, 410 U. S., at 139-140; id., at 176-177, n. 2 (Rehnquist, J., dissenting). On this record, it can scarcely be said that any deeply rooted tradition of relatively unrestricted abortion in our history supported the classification of the right to abortion as 'fundamental' under the Due Process Clause of the Fourteenth Amendment.*

*"We think, therefore, both in view of this history and of our decided cases dealing with substantive liberty under the Due Process Clause, that the Court was mistaken in Roe when it classified a woman's decision to terminate her pregnancy as a "fundamental right" that could be abridged only in a manner which withstood 'strict scrutiny.' In so concluding, we repeat the observation made in Bowers v. Hardwick, 478 U. S. 186 (1986):*

*'Nor are we inclined to take a more expansive view of our authority to discover new fundamental rights imbedded in the Due Process Clause. The Court is most vulnerable and comes nearest to illegitimacy when it deals with judge-made constitutional law having little or no cognizable roots in the language or design of the Constitution." Id., at 194.'*

*"We believe that the sort of constitutionally imposed abortion code of the type illustrated by our decisions following Roe is inconsistent 'with the notion of a Constitution cast in general terms, as ours is, and usually speaking in general principles, as ours does.' Webster v. Reproductive Health services, 492 U. S. at 518 (plurality opinion). The Court in Roe reached too far when it analogized the right to abort a fetus to the rights involved in Pierce, Meyer, Loving, and Griswold, and thereby deemed the right to abortion fundamental."*[13]

One of the most telling passages in the opinion of Kennedy, O'Connor, and Souter is where they essentially say that if they were to find Roe in error, the Court's reputation and power would be in doubt. Never mind that Roe might, indeed, have been in error. They just don't want to say so because their collective intellectual pride might be damaged, as would the legitimacy and power of this illustrious institution, the Supreme Court.

This is how the trio put it in their separate opinion:

*"If the Court's legitimacy should be undermined, then, so would the country be in its very ability to see itself through the*

*constitutional ideals. The Court's concern with legitimacy is not for the sake of the Court but for the sake of the Nation to which it is responsible.*

*The Court's duty in the present case is clear. In 1973, it confronted the already-divisive issue of governmental power to limit personal choice to undergo abortion, for which it provided a new resolution based on the due process guaranteed by the Fourteenth Amendment. Whether or not a new social consensus is developing on that issue, its divisiveness is no less today than in 1973, and pressure to overrule the decision, like pressure to retain it, has grown only more intense. <u>A decision to overrule Roe's essential holding would address error, if error there was, at the cost of both profound and unnecessary damage to the court's legitimacy,</u> and to the Nation's commitment to the rule of law. It is therefore imperative to adhere to the essence of Roe's original decision, and we do so today."*[14] (emphasis mine)

Blackmun and the majority of the justices based much of their decision on *stare decisis*, that rule of law that gives much weight to prior case law.

In other words, even if there had been error in Roe v. Wade, which has allowed millions of unborn babies to die legally, they wouldn't want to say so because it could damage their sacrosanct reputations. The minority opinion of Chief Justice Rehnquist and Justices Scalia, Thomas, and White, however, clearly says that if there is a question of an unsound decision at an earlier time, the Court must address that decision again.

*"Our constitutional watch does not cease merely because we have spoken before on an issue; when it becomes clear that a prior constitutional interpretation is unsound we are obliged to reexamine the question..."*

*"And, surely there is no requirement, in considering whether to depart from stare decisis in a constitutional case, that a decision be more wrong now than it was at the time it was rendered. If that were true, the most outlandish constitutional decision could survive forever, based simply on the fact that it was no more outlandish later than it was when originally rendered."*[15]

In order for women and their doctors to continue to have such preemptive rights over unborn children, the Court must continue to define the fetus as a non-person, undeserving of legal protection, and so they do. Just as in the Dred Scott decision, a black man was considered property, so are our pre-born children.

Just as the denial of the right to life for German Jews (and eventually anyone who was perceived to be the enemy of the State,) led to legal genocide in the Holocaust, so has Roe v. Wade.

The mental gymnastics needed to support abortion *in* Roe v. Wade, and now in Planned Parenthood v. Casey by those justices who did so, are difficult to comprehend. I think some of the decisions were pro-active, as in the case of Blackmun. And, I think some were results of intellectual pride, as in the case of Souter, Kennedy, and O'Connor, who need to "protect" the Court. The carefulness that they try to project in their convoluted writings only conceals the truth for a time. Hopefully, one day American citizens will take back their rights to make laws to protect unborn children.

Women are not freed by abortion, just as they are not enslaved by motherhood. Unborn babies are humans and deserve the protection of their right to life, liberty, and the pursuit of happiness.

When any of us loses his right to life, then we are all at risk. If there is such little regard for human beings in their most vulnerable stage of development, how much respect will there be for the older person who no longer is a productive entity, and may be very inconvenient to his or her family or to the State? How long before handicapped individuals are not respected and seen only as a burden? When expediency becomes our only criterion for protection of human life, then God help us!

If Blackmun, et al, want to continue the error that was Roe v. Wade, by striking down even the minimal protection that was passed by the State of Pennsylvania, then they will have to continue with rationalizations and penumbras that emanate from nowhere, and, if O'Connor, et al, want to continue the lie because the integrity of the Court would be damaged by admitting error, then we are all at risk. These kinds of entanglements in human thought and decisions can only further alienate humans, one from the other, and further erode the sanctity of human life.

---

[1] Joseph Sobran, *Single Issues*, The Human Life

Press, NY, 1983, p. *iv*.
[2] Supreme Court of the United States Syllabus, Planned Parenthood of Southeastern Pennsylvania et al, v. Casey, Governor of Pennsylvania, et al., Daily Appellate Report, Tuesday, June 30, 1992.
[3] Ibid.,p. 8982.
[4] Ibid., p. 9008.
[5] Ibid., p. 9004.
[6] Ibid.
[7] Ibid.
[8] Ibid., P. 9012.
[9] from *Fact Sheet*, "Abortion and Waiting Period Requirements," prepared by the Alan Guttmacher Institute for Planned Parenthood Federation of America, Inc. (FS-All, Rev. 1/93).
[10] Ibid.
[11] Ibid.
[12] Supreme Court of the United States Syllabus, Planned Parenthood of Southeastern Pennsylvania et al.,v. Casey, Governor of Pennsylvania, et al., Daily Appellate Report, Tuesday, June 30, 1992, p.9011.
[13] Ibid., pp. 9011, 9012.
[14] Ibid., p. 8991.
[15] Ibid, p. 9012.

# *A World Upside Down*

> "When we consider that women are treated as property, it is degrading to women that we should treat our children as property to be disposed of as we wish."
> _____Elizabeth Cady Stanton[1]

How did we get from legal protection for pre-born children to abortion as a necessity? Originally, even feminists considered abortion abhorrent, a travesty, the taking of a human life.

Margaret Sanger, a feminist, and the founder of Planned Parenthood, used an ad in 1916 for her first birth control clinic that stressed the need for contraception and the avoidance of the destruction of human life by abortion:

> *"Mothers, can you afford to have a large family? Do you want any more children? If not, why do you have them? Do not kill. Do not take life, but prevent. Safe, harmless information can be obtained of trained nurses at 46 Amboy Street, near Pitkin Ave., Brooklyn. Tell your friends and neighbors. All mothers welcome. A registration fee of 10 cents entitles any mother to this information."*[2]

Indeed, when Margaret Sanger was a nurse, she said,

> *"To see a baby born is one of the greatest experiences that a human being can have. Birth, to me, has always been more awe-inspiring than death. As often as I have witnessed the miracle, held the perfect creature with its tiny hands and tiny feet, each time I have felt as though I were entering a cathedral with prayer in my heart."*[3]

Eventually, however, Margaret Sanger found that abortion was a convenient way to deal with unplanned, unwanted pregnancies if contraception failed. In 1942, her organization, The American Birth Control League changed its name to Planned Parenthood, and it has since become the largest abortion provider in this country. Although it is supposed to be a non-profit organization, Planned Parenthood and its affiliates, as noted in the Preface to *Margaret Sanger, an Autobiography*,[4] had total budgets of about fifteen million dollars in 1970. I'm sure, with federal and corporate funding, their coffers are even larger now.

# A World Upside Down

The blueprints for the modern arguments for legal abortion were presented at a conference hosted by the National Committee on Maternal Health in 1942. Marvin Olasky detailed their proposals in his book, *The Press and Abortion, 1838-1988*. Here is his account of that conference.

*"Also, in 1942 the National Committee on Maternal Health held a conference on abortion at the New York Academy of Medicine and proposed four ways of handling the public relation problems that a pro-abortion position presented. First, Sophia Kleegman charged that restrictions on abortion were 'formulated largely by the <u>"theological dogma" of one "particular church.</u>"' Second, conference speakers argued that when abortion was a possibility for a woman, '<u>the ultimate decision should be hers.</u>' Third, conference speakers emphasized the desirability of <u>national uniformity</u> in abortion and proposed a model abortion law which could be accepted by all the states of this country. Fourth, Algernon Black of the Ethical Culture Society returned to the medically discredited 'quickening' distinction when he opposed the view that 'abortion is the destruction of a human being,' and other speakers followed along that line. Black contended that '<u>an unborn child has not the selfhood [sic], the relationships, or the consciousness of human personality-save potentially.</u>'"* [5] (emphasis added)

These same arguments are still used (sometimes in very creative ways) by pro-abortion activists. Their absolute implementation of these goals has been phenomenal and frightening. Especially effective has been the argument that a pre-born child does not have "selfhood" or "personhood."

At this point in time, when might a "non-person," the unborn child, be protected by law? Let's look at a few pending cases involving possible "fetal murder." There has been in California, recently, criminal prosecution that may eventually test the validity of the unborn child's personhood. The following is from the *Los Angeles Times*.

*"In what may be the first case of its kind in Los Angeles County, prosecutors filed murder charges Wednesday in the death of an 8-to 12-week-old fetus whose mother was injured in a gang-related shooting. A young woman was wounded and her unborn child killed in a drive-by shooting in the San Fernando Valley. The gang members, who*

> *assaulted her with gunfire, killed one other and wounded three of her friends, as they stood outside of an apartment building. Prosecutors charged the five alleged gang members with "fetus murder". Legal groundwork for the charge was paved in May by a California appellate court that ruled that every fetus is protected, regardless of its ability to sustain life outside the womb.*[6]

This is from the Los Angeles *Daily News*.

> *"Viability does not have to be an element of fetal murder,' said Deputy District Attorney Farnco Baratta, who filed the murder charge ...' "Baratta said he was able to file the fetal-murder charge in light of the 4th District Court of Appeal ruling that held that fetuses of all ages may be victims in murder cases." In People vs. Davis, however, the court held that prosecutors need only show that the fetus has progressed beyond 'embryonic stage' of seven or eight weeks for purposes of a murder charge, Baratta said.*[7]

This ruling, concerning an unborn child who was not considered "viable" at the time its life was ended by senseless violence, was based on another recent ruling in California that stated that even a non-viable fetus has a right to the state's protection. In 1991 in San Diego, in an armed robbery, a felon was convicted of murder and sentenced to life imprisonment for killing an unborn child. His mother survived, miraculously, a bullet in her chest. Her baby had been 25 weeks old.

In another case,

> *"Sherri Foreman, another victim of senseless violence, died as a result of her stabbing in another San Fernando Valley location in March of 1993. Her unborn child also died. She was attempting to withdraw money from an automated teller, when she was attacked. Her attacker will, of course, be tried for her murder, but the special circumstance of her 13- week-old unborn child may be used in the prosecution."*[8]

Why are these cases significant in regard to the continued legality of abortion? The Supreme Court, in a raw use of power ruled that the right of privacy gives a woman the right to kill her unborn child for any number of reasons--her physical or mental health (which usually means maintaining her present lifestyle), age, not wanting to raise a handicapped child, rape, or a lack of

# A World Upside Down

financial stability, to name a few. But, if someone else takes the life of her child it is a homicide. Why isn't it simply an illegal abortion?

The significance of these cases of fetal murder is explained by Anne Kindt, Attorney, and Executive Director of the Right to Life League of Southern California,

> *"It's a recognition that what resides in the womb is a person. It has to raise the question in people's minds: If we're prosecuting a third party for killing an unborn child, it's ironic a woman can choose an abortion for a child at that same date and we can't call it murder."*[9]

The importance of these and similar cases is not the question that a crime was committed, but how they will be prosecuted. Will the unborn fetus' right to life and protection by our laws be upheld? Or will the unclear thinking that began with finding a right to privacy in our Constitution for abortion be used again to exonerate those who take the lives of unborn children in criminal actions, without the consent of their mothers?

Another lawyer, Abby J. Leibman, Executive Director of the Women's Law Center, was quoted later in a *Los Angeles Times'* article with the following statement,

> *"Any time you have a court giving sanction to the notion that a fetus is a viable human being, it gives ammunition to those who would exalt the rights of an incipient human being over that of a viable, living human woman."*[10]

A statement from another abortion proponent in this same article came from law professor Christine Littleton. She said,

> *"The more you engage in this fantasy--and it is a fantasy--of thinking of the fetus as a separate person, then it's possible to envision all kinds of horrendous encroachments on the woman."*[11]

Ah, here lies the crux of the matter! The notion that a woman has the right to abortion, preeminently, over her unborn child's right to life, could be seriously damaged. Littleton used the word *encroachment*. Conversely, it seems to be very apropos in this case because that's exactly what an abortion is--an encroachment, not of the woman's right to her lifestyle, but of the unborn child's right to life. What about the fetus' <u>*right to privacy*</u>, the right to continue his existence in his natural, pre-birth environment?

This is their fear: that the truth of the humanity of the unborn child, which includes personhood, should be acknowledged by law. The truth would force them to concede what abortion really is—the destruction of innocent, human beings.

I have heard at various times, Jews, who favor abortion, articulate their disdain of the comparison of the legality of abortion as mass infanticide with the Jewish Holocaust at the hands of the Nazis. They are insulted by the comparison.

I have also heard angry remarks when the similarities are presented between the Dred Scott decision and *Roe v. Wade*. That a black man was considered a non-person, his master's property, is unconscionable, but somehow it's just and moral that pre-born children are considered non-persons, the property of their mothers.

Don Feder, a syndicated columnist with the Boston Herald, wrote an article about this comparison.

> *"In his book, The American Holocaust, William Brennan notes the similarities between the Nazi death camps and abortion clinics, including streamlined procedures for the disposal of unwanted life, practitioners of death who pride themselves on professionalism, experimentation on victims, and the assurance that the killing is legally sanctioned.*
>
> *It's all too easy to dismiss the Nazis as madmen. Fanatics they were, but fanatics with a vision: that not all life should be preserved, that certain creatures only appear to be people but in fact were less than human and thus could and should be sacrificed for a higher humanity. If abortion advocates are uncomfortable with the analogy, that is nothing next to the discomfort of those who are so dehumanized."*[12]

I have often wondered why the Jew or the black man doesn't see the essential parallels, and why they are insulted by similarities cited in the Dred Scott decision and the Nazi Holocaust. Maybe, those who are insulted by these comparisons feel that if they were to agree that there are parallels, they would then find themselves consciously or unconsciously siding with racism or genocide when they agree with *Roe v. Wade* and legal abortion. It seems that their denial of the validity of comparing legal abortion with Dred Scott and the Holocaust is indicative of the fear that they might be identified with something monstrous: the legal recognition of black human beings as non-persons (and thereby a justification for them to be considered property), or legal genocide of a certain class of individuals because they are unwanted (Jews in Germany or inconvenient pre-born children). If a black man or woman were to agree to the similarities in the cases, and then decide that he or she agreed with legal abortion because pre-borns were not persons, their thinking would be inconsistent with their disapproval of the Dred Scott decision. If a Jewish man or woman agreed that there were similarities between abortion and the mass elimination of Jews in the Nazi Holocaust, he or she would become, retroactively, a participant in that Holocaust. I understand why they vehemently deny the comparisons, but, by the same token, I don't understand why they aren't actively fighting for the lives of individuals who aren't able to defend themselves.

Rabbi Daniel Lapin shed some light on the liberal Jewish community's sanction of abortion on a radio broadcast I heard on *Focus on the Family*. He said,

> *"The Holocaust is one more way that we Jews have found to be Jewish without God. ...Why, on earth would I want to dwell on this tragic and horrible episode in Jewish history? The answer is that it serves this very valuable function. If you are somebody who wants to retain a kind of ethnic and cultural connection with Judaism, but you don't want God around, then the holocaust is tailor-made because it lets you speak about the one instance in history when it seems that God hid his face. ...And so, there is great Jewish indignation at using the term holocaust for what we know to be an absolute massacre of the unborn in the United States, and the reason is because the organized structure of the Jewish community, the leadership of the Jewish community has almost trademarked the word holocaust, and regards its use in almost any other context, as an infringement of trademark rights."*[13]

Our world has truly been turned upside down. Black is

white, and white is black. A drive-by shooting of an unborn child may be punishable by law, but an abortionist's right to kill them, twenty to thirty per day, is protected by the same law! Women's right to travel, work, or educate themselves in the manner they are accustomed to takes preference over the right to life of their unborn children.

Why has legalized abortion proliferated? Why has it become an acceptable way of life (and death)? One of the answers is contained in the following statement by Dr. Dallas Willard, a professor at USC, (University of Southern California) as published in an interview for the magazine, *Focus on the Family*. He describes the beginning of the pleasure principle, "meism", and the comfort-zone mentality that our nation has embraced.

*"The 1960s were a rebellion against anything other than pleasure. If religion wants back in, it has to come in that way. In earlier times the pursuit of God was part of happiness. It was God, self-denial, discipline. Your feelings and desires were regarded as potentially dangerous and not to be trusted. Now it's flipped around and they say, "just fulfill them."*[14]

Our children's educators have become the leading promoters of these pleasure principles--either because of their own personal agendas, or because of the directives and restrictions placed on them by the powers-that-be, the "educrats" who equate moral behavior with religion, and, therefore, improper material for public classroom discussion. In answer to the question, "How did we get to this point in our education system?" Eadie Gieb, the Director of Parents and Students United, a Los Angeles-based children's advocacy group, says:

*"In the early '70s, public school classrooms became a testing ground for ideas that have placed a wedge between parents and children. Instead of assisting the parents to uphold high moral standards, children began to be psychologically programmed to question or reject what they were taught at home, and to replace it with politically-correct, but morally bankrupt philosophies."*[15]

# A World Upside Down

I fear that we are raising a generation of children at this very moment (and have been doing so for several decades) who haven't learned even the very basics of moral behavior or self-discipline. My fear is that we have gone so far in our relentless pursuit of pleasure and comfort that very few adults and almost no children will value the moral principles that our country was founded on (or even hear of them). They are daily inundated with values-free education. And, along with that, they are exposed to the coarsest of sexual language on television, at the movies, or on the radio. They can find daily doses of murders, explosions, torture, and general human carnage on television and in the movies. It's called "entertainment." Is it any wonder that these same children grow up with a view that human life is not worth much? Is it any wonder that they can't form true, lasting relationships with the opposite sex because they aren't able to find examples of it in loving, married relationships--neither in the media, nor in their own families?

In May of 1993, Rand Corporation, a well-known think-tank located in Santa Monica, was able to administer for the second year in a row, over the objections of many students, parents, and teachers, a detailed sex survey. Not only were the questions intrusive, but the promised anonymity was a joke. Students, in order for a comparison to be made between '92 and '93 were asked to give their birth dates, both parents' first initials, and the last two digits of their phone number. It wouldn't be too difficult to find out which student had answered a particular questionnaire.

If I were to object to my children receiving, reading or participating in such an offensive, intrusive survey as the prurient Rand sex piece, I could claim invasion of privacy, but I wouldn't get very far. When parents asked if they could read the questionnaire ahead of time, only with perseverance, in spite of bureaucratic roadblocks, were they allowed to view it, and then only in the presence of a Rand employee. They were not allowed to copy it or to take notes or remove any pages! Invasion of privacy seems only to apply to abortion and the Roe v. Wade decision.

Some of the questions from the boys' questionnaire were:

*32. ...During the past year how many different times did these activities occur? (d) A girl put her mouth on your penis until you ejaculated (came). (h) You put your penis in a boy's anus (butt) or a boy put his penis in your anus.*

*39. During the NEXT YEAR, how likely is it that if you have anal intercourse, you will use a condom?*

*41. Which sexual orientation best describes you? (heterosexual, bisexual, homosexual and not sure.)*

*54. If you went to the doctor, would you trust him or her to keep things secret, if you didn't want your parents to know. If you thought you might be sexually attracted to other boys?"*

This question was blatantly designed to encourage young people to seek help without parental knowledge. If enough students were to answer false on this one, I'm sure the "correct" answer would be circulated to these poor, ignorant students, et al.

In New York, school children were introduced to something called the "Children of the Rainbow" curriculum. One of the stories was "Heather has Two Mommies." By the fourth grade, students would learn all about oral and anal sex. Luckily, parents united under the leadership of School Board President, Mary Cummins. Not only did they succeed in ousting this curriculum, but they also ousted school chancellor Joseph Fernandez. The Children of the Rainbow series was dubbed "The Fernandez-Dinkins Pornographic Sex Guide". Mayor Dinkins was not re-elected, either.

# A World Upside Down

Black and white don't exist anymore--only rainbow colors (mommies and daddies of the same sex) are socially correct. When expediency replaces morality, as it does in abortion, and values-free sex education supplants the need for moral guidance for our young people, we have a world not only upside down, but lopsided as well, spinning at full-tilt in a shocking downward spiral. When the whirling finally stops, we will find that we have a culture based on high-tech utilitarianism, advanced by a people who have never experienced or been exposed to selflessness, self-discipline, courage, or respect for one another as fellow human beings.

---

[1] Elizabeth Cady Stanton, as cited by Randy Alcorn in *Pro Life Answers to Pro Choice Arguments*, Multnomah Books, Questar Publishers, Sisters, Oregon, 1992, p. 95. The quote is from a letter in Julia Ward Howe's Journal, 16 October 1873, available at Houghton Library, Harvard University.
[2] Marvin Olasky, *The Press and Abortion*, Lawrence Erblum Assoc., Hillsdale, N.J., 1988, p. 216.
[3] Margaret Sanger, *Margaret Sanger, an Autobiography*, Maxwell Reprint Co., NY 1970, p. 55.
[4] Ibid.
[5] Marvin Olasky, *The Press and Abortion*, Lawrence Erlbum Assoc. Hillsdale, NJ 1988, pp. 77 & 78.
[6] Leslie Berger, "Valley Case May Become test for 'Fetus Murder'," *Los Angeles Times*, June 20, 1993, A 21
[7] Los Angeles *Daily News*, June 17, 1993, front section, p. 3.
[8] Leslie Berger, "Valley Case May Become test for 'Fetus Murder', *Los Angeles Times*, June 20, 1993, A 21.
[9] Ibid..
[10] Ibid.
[11] Ibid.
[12] Don Feder, "Nazism and Abortion," in *All About Issues* magazine, March-April 1992, American Life League, Inc., Stafford Va., p. 14.
[13] Rabbi Daniel Lapin, from "Examining the Roots of Judeo Christian Values," a radio broadcast of *Focus on the Family*, Colorado Springs,

Co., April, 1996.

[14] Dallas Willard, "Why Is Everyone So Angry?," an interview of Dr. Willard of the University of Southern California, in *Focus on the Family Citizen Magazine*, Colorado Springs, Co., Vol 7, No. 5, May 17, 1993, pp. 14 & 15

[15] Eadie Gieb, from a personal interview by the author in August, 1993.

[16] Rand Corporation's "Sex Survey," Santa Monica, Ca., May 1993.

# Abortion & The Politically Correct

"In the matter of abortion the words of the Constitution did not change, but on January 22, 1973, its meaning did. On that date Justice Harry Blackmun found in the Ninth Amendment's reservation of power to the People or in the Fourteenth Amendment's reference to liberty--he was not entirely sure in which--a liberty to consent to an abortion. On that date the Constitution came to mean that abortion was an American freedom." _____ John Noonan[1]

President Clinton, at one point, in his "after-election campaigning," said that he would like to see abortions "safe, legal, and rare," and yet on January 22, 1993 he signed into law some of the most pro-abortion legislation since 1973. And, he has since campaigned for government funding of abortions, and for these elective procedures to be performed by military physicians for women in our armed forces. For him to say he wants abortions to become rare and then to support and promote the use of federal funds to help destroy our unborn citizens is not abortion-neutral. It's political double-talk. Clinton and his administration are also committed to easier access to abortion throughout the world. Their idea that we will save the world by killing unborn children on a grand scale is so unconscionable that it staggers the mind. They are asking for a strongly worded statement in favor of abortion at a United Nations population conference scheduled for 1994.

They seem to believe that population control, by way of freely offered and available abortion, is a *moral good.* They promote the idea that our planet will solve all of its population problems by making abortion acceptable, fashionable, and politically correct. Many of our young people *sincerely* believe this. This is what they have learned in their schools and in their homes.

Those who advocate abortion for purposes of limiting the world's population include some very well-known names: today, President Clinton; yesterday, Margaret Sanger.

How did the political climate become so favorable for legal abortion? The scare-tactics of over-population as an issue was quite effective in the sixties. Near the end of the decade and the beginning of the seventies, four political over-populationists were appointed by President Richard Nixon:

*"Within the executive branch, for example, Richard Nixon in*

*1969 and 1970, made four critical appointments that affected abortion policy. John Ehrlichman, who was pro-abortion, became domestic chief of staff; Louis Hellman, a director of the Association for the Study of Abortion, took the key spot for abortion policy in the Department of Health, Education, and Welfare; John D. Rockefeller III, who spoke for and heavily funded the pro-abortion forces, became chairman of a 'Commission on Population Growth and the American Future;' and Harry Blackmun became a Supreme Court justice. Although Nixon himself made a few politically useful anti-abortion comments, his administration included ardent pro-abortionists such as Reimer Ravenholt who helped to fund many pro-abortion conferences. Of Nixon's 20 appointees to the commission chaired by Rockefeller, 16 were pro-abortion, and it predictably recommended abolition of all abortion laws."*[1]

Mr. Clinton, also, has been pro-active on the issue of abortion, by way of some of his important presidential appointments. A politically-correct example is his choice for Surgeon-General, Dr. M. Joycelyn Elders. She believes in and actively promotes abortion, school-based clinics, and sex education for even the youngest of our children.

From an article in the *Los Angeles Times* about Elders, on March 8, 1993:

*"She has called fundamentalists opposed to abortion 'very religious non-Christians,' accused them of operating from a 'slave-master mentality' and once branded two of their leaders 'mean, ugly and evil.' "*[3]

Quoting Elders in the same Los Angeles Times article,

*" 'If Medicaid does not pay for abortions, does not pay for family planning, but pays for prenatal care and delivery, that's saying: 'I'll pay for you to have another good, healthy slave, but I won't pay for you to use your brain and make choices for yourself,' she explains.' "*[4]

This is disingenuous. Not paying for abortions or for contraceptives does not constitute government abandonment of needy individuals. No one would deny federal funds for a truly "life-saving" abortion.

Elders goes on in that article,

# Abortion & The Politically Correct

*"The public assistance tab for teen mothers and their children came to $26 billion in 1991, up from $19.3 billion four years earlier. Single, unemployed with no job skills and on welfare, children who have children constitute America's newest slave class..."[5]*

Why has "the tab for teen mothers and their children" become so much higher now? Haven't Planned Parenthood, et al, done their job with condoms in schools and promotion of abortion? Or has the push for "safe sex" led kids to believe that everyone does it, therefore it must be the thing to do? Why hasn't the tide of epidemic teen pregnancies been turned with this aggressive, amoral agenda?

It seems from what she says and from what she proposes that Mrs. Elders' plan is to ensure that children don't have children by first of all teaching them all about sex in the schools (taking this prerogative out of the hands of their parents), by offering contraceptives at school clinics, taking any suggestion of self-control or abstinence out of the picture, and then giving the State, its teachers and counselors, the right to "help" a teen have an abortion without her parents' knowledge.

It seems to me that all this freedom offered to our teen girls is a thinly disguised means of control devised by a pervasive government that thinks it knows better and has more rights to children's lives than their parents!

In the May 24 issue of Time magazine, Elders said:

*"We've allowed the right to make decisions about our children for the last 100 years, and all it has bought us is the highest abortion rate, the highest non-marital birth rate and the highest pregnancy rate in the industrialized world."[6]*

Very interesting! She said, "we've allowed." We've allowed whom? Parents? Since when do parents need to be allowed to raise their children? Since when does someone else know better than parents?

An editorial in the Los Angeles *Daily News* questioned this bizarre statement,

*"What exactly is Elders saying? If she thinks unfettered parental autonomy is to blame for the alarming increase in teen pregnancies and abortions, she has her culprits all wrong. Dramatic increases in those social pathologies have taken a sharp turn not in the 'last 100 years,' but in the past two or three decades, precisely the time when the public*

*schools have been encroaching on the parents' traditional role of conveying sexual knowledge and morality to children.'"*

I wonder if Elders realizes that if her ideology had been politically-correct in 1933, she probably would have been eliminated before she was born. She was conceived by a teen-age mother and a sharecropper father. I wonder if she understands that what she is promoting for others would have eliminated her right to live safely in her mother's womb, and then to be a young girl, a doctor, and, yes, even her right to be a mother. Certainly the timing of her birth couldn't have been optimum or planned! Certainly her parents and grandparents would have chosen the "responsible" decision of abortion.

Elders accused Christians who oppose abortion of operating from a slave-master mentality. Let's discuss what real slavery is--in the guise of "choice."

If a pregnant or sexually active teen girl goes to a school-based clinic or a counselor for help, she would have the choice of an abortion, contraceptives, including the pill and Norplant.

She isn't given the choice of learning about her own self-worth and dignity. She won't find in the classroom or in the school clinic the truth about the fact that she should say no to her boyfriend when he pressures her into a sexual relationship. Nor, will she hear from her teachers that there are a certain set of basic moral values that will promote a healthy, functioning, fulfilling life.

Any instruction that even appears to include values is labeled religious in nature. "Mrs. Smith, we can't teach Johnny that a casual, sexual relationship with three girls in his class could be wrong or immoral. You know that is a religious point of view." or "Oh, of course not, Mrs. Smith, we wouldn't teach Suzie that she should say no. We know it doesn't work, anyway. Besides we can't impose our values on your children." Of course, I'm paraphrasing what they might really, more politically-correctly say.

My nephew, who graduated from high school this past June, a basketball star and the valedictorian of his class, said that he is insulted by those who tell him that they know he isn't able to control himself, that "he's going to do it anyway," so he'd better learn "safe sex." I'll bet somewhere along the line he had a teacher who supported what his parents tried to instill in him. He has a steady girlfriend, and she feels the same way, too. Amazing! They find value in "saving themselves" for marriage and a committed relationship. They both have very full, active lives. They don't feel deprived. I predict that they will find freedom in their decision to wait for sex --rather than repression.

Values are not meant to be restrictive, nor are they. They are actually where our freedoms lie. When young men and women learn only unconstrained, values-free behavior under the label of "safe sex" they are not learning about freedom (or even about "safety"), but about self-centeredness and self-gratification which can become addiction and enslavement, as surely as drugs and alcohol enslave.

We are inherently moral creatures with a desire to form ourselves in some moral order, but we also are sinful creatures who seek pleasure without restraint. When we tell ourselves that the sin of promiscuity is our own private business, (a victimless crime) the results hurt us, our families, and society. Those who would teach children that they have to make up their own minds, "responsibly," about having sexual experiences at the ages of 12, 13, or 14 are doing them no favors, nor society either.

In my experience with young people over the last twenty years in the counseling center, we have seen the results of sex education served up in our schools. It has caused confusion, at the very least, and heartache, ultimately, in the lives of our children! When they seek guidance from their teachers and counselors, they are given how-to pictures of sexual intercourse.

Unfortunately, Elders and her agenda is in. Those who would ask young people to be responsible and abstinent until marriage are out. The result will be more children having children and more abortions for any reason, at any time.

Those who believe that abortion should be legal give the argument that women have always gotten abortions anyway, legally or illegally. At least, with legal abortion, it will be safe, they say. Women won't lose their lives or be damaged from legal abortions. It's true that abortions would still be sought and found if abortion were illegal. But, not on the scale of a million and a half a year (approximately 4,400 per day). Has anyone ever wondered where the illegal abortionists from the back alleys have gone? Would it be reasonable to assume that they have just moved to the front now? Would it be reasonable to assume that their methods are not much different, not much safer in light of the high-volume of procedures done in one day?

I counseled a woman the other day who was determined to have an abortion, no matter what. Molly had never wanted children, and there would be no discussion now. She was concerned, however, about her own safety. I told her to make sure that wherever she went the doctor was reliable and known to be safe. Molly went that day to a local clinic for her abortion. I talked to her after the procedure, and she told me that when she "dared" to ask the abortionist about his medical license and malpractice insurance, he said, "Get out of here." But, because the clinic looked okay to her, she had her abortion there anyway. I guess he was willing to forgive her and take her cash, even though she had insulted him.

Women who have their babies and choose to raise them most often become responsible mothers. They think more than twice about getting pregnant again. They will either establish a permanent relationship with the father of their child (possibly by marriage) or they will dissolve the relationship and be more careful before getting involved again in a relationship that could lead to more unintended pregnancies. In other words, caring for the child she gave birth to makes her more aware of the consequences of her actions and more responsible before she skips merrily into another sexual relationship.

The woman who would not consider having an abortion if it were illegal would be better off. She would not have to bear the grief and guilt that comes with the loss of her son or daughter. The child, of course, will be better off--he has been given life. And, society itself will gain from men and women who learn that their actions have consequences, that "quick fixes" to long-term problems don't work. Often, I have asked women who were seeking an abortion what they would do if it were illegal. Strangely enough, most of them think of alternatives. Only a few have said that they would seek an illegal abortion.

I say to the over-populationists that the idea that more abortions equals fewer people is wrong. A majority of women I have spoken to over the years will have another child soon after the first or second abortion. Consciously or unconsciously they try to get pregnant in order to make up for the death of children who were lost in the abortions. There might be fewer mouths to feed because of abortion, but there possibly could be more.

The same individuals and organizations who promote abortion for purposes of population control, will use every means available to promote environmental protection for even the lowliest creatures--the snail darter, (whatever that is) among them. We must save the whales and the spotted owl. How about the cheetah and the rain forests? What about the family of man, the pre-born babies?

The amount of time and public funds spent on the California condor is an example of politically-correct priorities.

# Abortion & The Politically Correct

The poor bird has been forced to live and breed in captivity so that it doesn't become extinct. Has anyone ever thought that maybe the condor's time has come and gone? That, possibly, it doesn't need man's interference to prolong its continued existence? Evolution and subsequent extinction could be the natural order of things. Then again, maybe left in its own natural habitat with its own methods of procreation it might survive and thrive.

Certainly our world, with its beautiful rivers, oceans, and forests, needs to be protected, but without basic protection and respect for humanity, it means nothing. Spotted owls are in, pre-born baby humans are out!

What is the connection between the environmentalists and the abortion lobby? I really wasn't able to figure it out for many years. Daniel Lapin spoke about this connection on that same radio broadcast of *Focus on the Family* that I mentioned in Chapter 3. Rabbi Lapin said,

> *"It is part of our function in drawing closer to God, that we separate ourselves from the animal world. ...What on earth do radical environmentalists have to do with the homosexual rights movement? ...Why is it that they have Sex Ed in school, which is nothing other than an indoctrination machine to strip young people of their natural God-given modesty? Why don't we have Weapons Ed? Why don't we say that if they're going to use them, they might as well know how to use them safely? ...The radical environmentalists' agenda is an attempt to strip the first few chapters of Genesis from the Bible. It is an indication of the ascending order of importance in creation. What is undeniably clear is that human beings are not just another form of animals."*[8]

And, if we deny those chapters in the Bible, we can deny the immorality of homosexual relationships. We will be able to take God and his divine order of creation out of our lives, so that we will have more choices.

It is a political lie that those who promote abortion are promoting "choice." There are many examples, besides Pennsylvania, of individual states attempting to "choose" to place some protection for the unborn in their laws. Those who promote legal abortion, like Planned Parenthood, don't want individual states to have a real choice--one that might restrict abortion in any way.

A very frightening piece of legislation has been making the rounds for the last few years that would deny the possibility of any pro-life legislation that might dare to appear in any individual state. Pro-abortionists devised (just in case) legislation that would be a *be-all* and *end-all* answer if, indeed, Roe were ever reversed. The so-called Freedom of Choice Act has been introduced in the House of Representatives and the Senate. I first heard about this possible legislation in 1991. The analyses of the bill presented by several different attorneys, political scientists and law professors, were breathtaking. Because of the simplicity and breadth of the proposed legislation, no laws could ever be passed in any state that would offer any protection for the unborn child. If Roe can be described as abortion on demand, with the possibility of parole, then F.O.C.A. (the Freedom of Choice Act) can be described as the death penalty for the unborn, without the possibility of even an appeal. No states could write laws that would limit abortions for any reason, other than the health of the mother.

I wrote a letter to both California senators, Dianne Feinstein and Barbara Boxer, regarding the Freedom of Choice Act. I received a form letter back from both. Feinstein stated that "...states may still enact their own laws to protect unwilling persons from participating in abortion procedures if it is contrary to their moral or religious belief, decline funding of procedures and require the involvement of parents, guardians or other responsible adults in the abortion decision of minors..."

Either Feinstein is sadly ill-informed, doesn't understand the scope of the simple language, or she seeks to assuage her constituency with political newspeak. The Freedom of Choice Act, introduced by Rep. Don Edwards, (D-Cal) states quite simply and very broadly the following, from Section 2 of the bill:

*"(a) In general--except as provided in subsection (b), a State may not restrict the right of a woman to choose to terminate a pregnancy (1) before fetal viability; or (2) at any time, if such termination is necessary to protect the life or health of the woman. Subsection (b) Medically Necessary Requirements--A state may impose requirements medically necessary to protect the life or health of women referred to in subsection (a)."*

In other words, states could not place any restrictions on abortion unless the health or life of the mother would be threatened by that abortion. The F.O.C.A. would invalidate all restrictions now imposed in any state or any restrictions that might be desired in the future, including rights that the State might now have in place to regulate abortions in the third trimester.

Boxer said in her form letter: "Section 3 of the Freedom

of Choice Act states that nothing in the Act can 'prevent a State from requiring a minor to involve a parent, guardian, or *other responsible* (emphasis added) adult before terminating a pregnancy." The key term here is that "any responsible adult" can take anyone's precious minor child to an abortionist without the knowledge of that child's parents or guardian! How is responsibility determined? A minor girl's adult boyfriend could take her for an abortion (What else is new?), or a school counselor, or an older friend (age 18 or 21?) would do.

Another "freedom" that would result from F.O.C.A.. would be the legal right to hire medical personnel, other than doctors, to perform abortions. In other words, a trained technician, midwife, or whoever, would be able to perform the procedure. As it is now, abortion clinics and their doctors are one of the least regulated medical services in our country, and this added license of abortion-by-technician will expand the atrocities practiced on desperate women. <u>The only difference between an illegal abortion of 25 years ago and a legal abortion after F.O.C.A. would be the terminology.</u>

States would not be able to require parental notification or consent. They could not legislate for a 24-hour waiting period. Currently, abortion is the only medical procedure where the physician is not required to present full information about the procedure or about fetal development. In fact, when an ultrasound is needed to determine the age of the unborn, it is turned from the view of the pregnant woman. If she is quite sure of her abortion decision, shouldn't she see what the "products of conception" look like before they are extracted?

Whether or not this comprehensive, pro-abortion bill becomes law at this time remains to be seen. But if it does, America's women will once again be the losers. Safe, legal abortion will become a fast-food industry--in fact, a service offered without the inspections, regulations, or safeguards that are necessary to operate a McDonald's or a Taco Bell.

Roe v. Wade has appeared, at different times, to be threatened in the last few years by various cases being heard by the Supreme Court.

As discussed in the last chapter, *Planned Parenthood, et al*, brought a class action suit against Governor Robert Casey and Pennsylvania because they had had the audacity to sign into law some minor limits on abortion. In the final ruling, the Supreme Court let stand some restrictions and struck down others, thereby reaffirming Roe v. Wade, but not specifically forbidding states to make some laws about abortion regulation.

In March of 1993, Governor Casey gave a speech in the historic old Courthouse in St. Louis where the original Dred Scott trial was held. He opened his remarks by referring to his political position within his own Democratic party. He had been denied the right to speak (Talk about choice and political correctness!) at the 1992 Democratic National Convention.

*"As I discovered, even the governor of a major state who holds pro-life views can be denied a hearing at his party's convention without the national media protesting it."*[9] (emphasis added)

Casey quoted some of his fellow Democrats in a speech he gave to the Notre Dame Law School on April 2, 1992.

*"Three years ago, Speaker of the House Tom Foley assured reporters that there was no formal Democratic leadership position on abortion. My, how times have changed. Just listen to what he gratuitously declared in his response to the President's State of the Union address. Even though the President made no mention of abortion, for some reason Foley could not resist issuing this prediction to the national television audience: 'If the Supreme Court removes the guarantees of choice from the Constitution of the United States, this Congress will write it into the laws of the United States.'"* [10]

Another Democrat quoted by Casey said, in 1977,

*"What happens to the mind of a person, and the moral fabric of a nation, that accepts the aborting of the life of a baby without a pang of conscience? What kind of a person, what kind of a society, will we have 20 years hence if life can be taken so casually?"*[11]

This was a statement made by Reverend Jesse Jackson four years after Roe v. Wade. His need to be politically-correct has changed his viewpoint since then. But his question about our society, unfortunately, will read like prophecy in 1997, unless some exceptional changes in the pro-life direction occur very soon.

Thomas Jefferson, the founder of the Democratic Party, wrote over two hundred years ago, "We hold these Truths to be self-evident, that all men are created equal, that they are endowed by their Creator with certain unalienable Rights, that among these are Life, Liberty and the Pursuit of Happiness..." I guess his party now has decided only liberty and the pursuit of happiness have validity. The unalienable right to life is questionable.

Governor Casey also spoke about some of the ugly pro-abortion tactics that were used when he ran for reelection in 1990,

> "Pro-choice groups sent several dozen of their supporters to the Governor's Residence, where they chanted, 'Get your rosaries off my ovaries,' as the television cameras whizzed. And my opponent, who spent $2 million, dramatized my position of refusing to recognize an exception for rape by running a television commercial that purported to depict a rape, and in which it was difficult to distinguish me from the rapist."[12]

This sophomoric, politically-correct chant and the rapist political spot must come from very misguided, very angry individuals, and is difficult even to comment on. It is so tasteless, so ludicrous, that it leaves one speechless.

I heard "get your rosaries off my ovaries" for the first time several years ago at the Her Medical (abortion) Clinic in Pacoima, California, where pro-life demonstrators were blocking the clinic entrance in protest. Both Barbara Boxer (then a California U. S. representative) and Gray Davis (California's Controller) joined a pro-abortion crowd with bull horns. As they played the crowd, (which included masked mimes carrying crucifixes affixed with Barbie dolls entwined in rosaries) I stood next to them. To say that they behaved in an undignified manner is to say the very least. They used their bull horns to encourage and hype the mimes and the crowd. Their blocking of the street and their freedom of speech was upheld, correctly, by many police officers. Mine, however, was not.

I had been told by a policeman that they could stand in the street, which was off-limits to the protesters and to me, because "*they* were somebody", which, of course, implied that I was nobody, and did not have the same rights to freedom of speech. So, I *lawfully* , silently prayed for them as they cheered on the repulsive show.

Casey challenges the argument that some hold: that we must bring about change by persuasion, not coercion i. e., legal restraint. Since when are laws prohibiting the destruction of human beings coercive or religious? To refrain from killing for moral reasons, or in the interests of an ordered society, is not unique to religious institutions and their members. And, even if it were only "religious" people who subscribed to a moral code that excluded the killing of pre-born humans, it wouldn't negate the truth of the immorality and unacceptability of the act. I have heard many, even those who claim to be pro-life, say that we must change people's hearts and minds—that changing the law or amending the Constitution is not what's needed. When Roe v. Wade came into existence by decree of seven men, it changed the hearts and minds of future generations. By casting abortion as a legal right, it implied that it is a *moral good*. If we don't turn back to the source of this evil and change it, it will be impossible to change people *one heart and mind at a time*.

The Hyde Amendment, which prohibits use of federal funds for abortions, has often been under attack, as has its author, Representative Henry Hyde of Illinois. In 1977, a year after this amendment had been passed, the American Civil Liberties Union (ACLU), Planned Parenthood, and others joined forces to oppose the ban. They were able to find a federal judge who enjoined the enforcement of the amendment. Mr. Hyde details what happened next in his book, *For Every Idle Silence*.[13] Part of their strategies in the case included a theory put forth that the:

> *"...Hyde Amendment 'used the fist of government to smash the wall of separation between church and state by imposing a peculiarly religious view of when a human life begins.' To gather support for this theory, the plaintiffs asked <u>to review my mail in order to find expressions of religious sentiment</u>..."*[14]
>
> *"So the plaintiffs' lawyers and my lawyers sat down and examined great piles of my mail. They did find expressions of religious sentiment. The ACLU and Planned Parenthood lawyers drew up a large chart. Whenever they found a letter that supported my view on abortion and closed with an expression such as 'God bless you,' one of the lawyers solemnly checked an appropriate box on the chart with further evidence of a religious conspiracy."*[15]

If a politician were trying to promote laws that would force people to engage in, or be restricted by, something that is uniquely a religious practice, they would most definitely be coercive and acting outside of the Constitution. That would truly be the State imposing a religious view on its citizens. But when basic human morality is portrayed as exclusively a religious law, then we are caught in a tangle of illogical rhetoric. Morality, whether it be explicitly stated in the ten commandments or implicitly written on the hearts and minds of men is a fact of human existence. It does, indeed, separate us from the animal kingdom.

The former Mayor of New York, Ed Koch, once wrote in a column that he supports Roe v. Wade and abortion wholeheartedly, even though he acknowledges that sometime, possibly after the first trimester, it is infanticide.[16] He supports the killing of unborn children wholeheartedly, even when he acknowledges the fact that it is infanticide?!! I don't know why I still find statements like these shocking.

In reply to a high school student's question (in Chillicothe, Ohio) about abortion, President Clinton said that almost all Americans oppose legal abortion when children can live outside their mother's womb. "When children" is the key phrase here because he acknowledged that they are children whether *in utero* or *ex utero*. It's only a matter of location! Will this little matter of location mean someday that my personhood depends on whether I must live at a hospital in order to survive, or whether I can live outside the hospital (the womb) on my own?

There are those who will not say children, as Clinton 'mistakenly' did, but who promote the blob theory when referring to the unborn child. The notion that the fetus is only a blob at the time of an abortion can't even be defended realistically by an abortionist. If a woman tries to get an abortion soon after she finds out she's pregnant, which might be only twelve days after conception, she will be told to wait for four or five more weeks. The reason for this is that the unborn child must be large enough to protrude from the uterine wall, so as not to be missed by the abortionist's knife. The abortion is a blind procedure, and if the child is left in the uterus, infection may occur or an unhealthy pregnancy may continue. At six weeks, the child's heart has been beating since the eighteenth day and brain waves can be detected. The unborn child only becomes a blob after the vacuum aspiration procedure. In later abortions, around twelve weeks, the abortionist needs to identify all of the body parts to be sure that the unborn baby's arms and legs, trunk, head, and torso have all been extracted from its mother's uterus. These are not politically-correct images to broadcast to the general public-- but they are the facts.

When those who are pro-abortion debate the issue, they very carefully leave out many of these facts. They prefer to use the term, *fetus*, which sounds less human. Sometimes, when challenged, they opt for the truth because they have no other recourse.

The following dialogue is excerpted from a call-in Talk

Show, *Live from L. A.*, on KKLA /FM, here in Southern California, on June 4, 1993. It is not verbatim, but the essence of the participants' stands on different issues remains. Jack Kocienski hosted the program. His guests were Mary Hunt, of Women's Alliance For Theology, Ethics and Ritual and of Catholics for a Free Choice, and Matt Spalding of the Claremont Institute, here in California.

*Jack: <u>Do you think abortion is the taking of a human Life?</u>*

*Mary: That's not the language I would use.*

*Matt: A pregnancy creates a human life.*

*Jack: <u>How do you feel about natural law?</u>*

*Mary: Social justice tradition, seeing abortion in the concrete. I see it in light of each woman. The more contemporary social justice position is that we are starting at a different point. Many of us who are Catholic differ with the Church on its teaching on abortion. There should be an eradication for the need of the choice of abortion.*

*Matt: Natural law was put forward by Catholic theologians, but it is not really a Catholic teaching--it's a common-sense idea.*

*Jack: Natural laws are standards of justice inherent in what we are. If you understand what a human being is, then you understand that he has the right to live. (Jack cited the Declaration of Independence, and the Nuremburg Trials.) <u>Please comment.</u>*

*Matt: Laws should be based on a common sense of justice, which is based on nature. The ground of individualism must be in nature. (He cited slavery along with abortion.)*

*Mary: It's a nice part of our history, but it's rather anachronistic to have recourse to natural law. (She's astonished at his answer because her Washington think tanks have not for a long time referred to natural law. She opposes the death penalty quite strongly.) It's preposterous to say that Thomas Aquinas is the greatest theologian in the Catholic church. I hope that we would agree within the Christian community that the death penalty is an egregious violation of natural law or contextual ethics (her term).*

# Abortion & The Politically Correct

*Matt:* I believe that abortion is the central question to those group of issues we generally describe when we talk about cultural issues. You mentioned the Washington think tanks. I think that the tradition of the natural law is not outdated (he cites Clarence Thomas' nomination and the natural law questions). The think tanks don't respond to natural law--all they know and espouse is moral relativism.

*Jack:* <u>But, what about human life, in plain English?</u>

*Mary:* In plain English, abortion is ending a pregnancy. A woman begins pregnant, she has an abortion, she's no longer pregnant. I am pro-choice, I start as a feminist with a pregnant woman and I regret every time a woman who is pregnant has to make a decision to have an abortion. This is a regrettable, tragic problem every time it happens, but I do not consider it immoral, nor do I think it should be illegal, nor do I think it should be expensive, and yes I think it is something the government should pay for.

*Jack:* <u>Is it tragic for both the woman and the child that is aborted?</u>

*Mary:* I don't consider it's a child that's aborted. I will not have words put in my mouth. The word child is not one that I will use. I use an embryo, a pre-embryo, or a fetus.

*Jack:* <u>I don't feel you've answered my question.</u>

*Mary:* I believe in the work of Professor Clifford Grothstein of how a pre-embryo becomes an embryo, becomes a fetus, and eventually becomes a child. You and I would agree that abortion earlier in the process from conception to the experience of birth and neo-natalhood for a child would argue for having an early abortion.

*Jack:* <u>Don't put words in my mouth. I will not agree with that. It's murder from day one.</u>

*Radio Listener/Caller:* I encouraged my wife to have an abortion over 14 years ago. I anguish over this, as does my wife who has a hidden hurt.

*Mary:* The Catholic church has never baptized the material that results in miscarriage. One doesn't engage in Baptism because this isn't a *person.*

*Matt: If the child is in the process of being born, it can be baptized. The point about defining terms is a very academic use, and the ethicists like to call things what they're not.*

*Mary: Let's agree with the terms that the in utero material is, of course, human. There's no question there's something there that is alive. What we disagree on is personhood. I would not make the claim that the value of what is in utero three days after conception and three days after birth is the same. Many of the mainline Christian denominations do have pro-choice stands.*

*Brad Listener/Caller: Where do you draw a line, if at all, right before the birth, or five months after conception? And if you think abortion is OK, why don't we show the American public what it's really like? Why not on television?*

*Mary: I don't think that abortion is no big deal. But for a woman to have an abortion is not in fact a source of scandal or something she needs to be ashamed of either. Because there are circumstances. I trust women to make good moral choices. I have known women who have chosen abortion. Why not have it on TV? I don't think that this is a problem. I think that people shouldn't be squeamish. I do not consider this more than a medical procedure. I don't think the truth hurts. Nobody likes abortion. I am not one who draws a line anywhere, and it is not up to me to draw the line. It exists in the context of the woman. It does not exist by itself. At the time of birth there are two people. Until then, there is a pregnant woman and her part of the moral equation is important.*

*Kathy Listener/Caller: My husband and I have gone through in vitro fertilization three times. Three days after my egg and my husband's sperm are fertilized they make an embryo, they are now four cells. The doctor will wheel them into the room where I am ready to have my uterus implanted. They are in an incubator. The room is darkened, voices are asked to be hushed because these real embryos are sensitive to light and sound. Why is it if you want the child it's a life, but when it's inconvenient it's not a life?*

*Mary: But it's not a person.*

*Matt: Well, then, what is a person?*

*Mary: Personhood is conferred not at the moment of conception, but when there are certain other criteria: ability to enter a relationship and the individuation...*

*Kathy: In 1970, when I was pregnant, I went to nuns and priests, who said abortion was the way to go. I am now not able to have children. You did me no favors.*[17]

I present this debate, not for its scholarship, but rather because it is a good example of the social and political debate as it stands now in our nation.

Those who are politically incorrect, such as Henry Hyde or Governor Robert Casey, Representative Chris Smith, or Senators Orrin Hatch and Strom Thurmond, to name just a few, are our real statesmen. They, and others like them, hopefully, will stand between our nation's survival and its demise as a free state, protecting even the most vulnerable individuals.

John Noonan, in his book, *A Private Choice*, discusses error and the Supreme Court:

> "...The Supreme Court can be wrong. What the Supreme Court says the Constitution means can do violence to every criterion of history and logic. Instead of developing the purposes of the framers, the Court can subvert them. The Supreme Court can find in the term "liberty" in the Fourteenth Amendment the liberty of a factory owner to work his employees more than ten hours a day, and the Court can be outrageously wrong in so finding. But the law of the land, the meaning of the Constitution as a legal document, will be what the Court says the meaning is, until it admits its error or is corrected by a constitutional amendment.
>
> "A decision of the Supreme Court, then, is the last word on the meaning of the Constitution--for the time being. The interpretation offered by the Court can last only as long as the Court is convinced that the interpretation is correct. The Court's conviction of its own correctness does not depend solely on its own precedents; otherwise there would be no change and no reversals of direction by the Court. Like it or not, the Court is engaged in an exchange with its critics, in which its critics always have the power to persuade the Court that it was wrong, or the power to persuade the President to appoint successor justices who believe the Court was wrong, or the power to persuade the country to adopt an amendment to the Constitution correcting the error of the

Court.[1]

Governor Casey, in his St. Louis speech, quoted Abraham Lincoln and his remarks about the need for some checks on the power of the Supreme Court:

*"In his first Inaugural address, Abraham Lincoln, in referring to the Dred Scott case, expressed the view that other officers of the government could not be obligated to accept any new laws created by the Court unless they, too, were persuaded by the force of the Court's reasoning. Any other position would mean, in his view, that 'the policies of the government upon vital questions, affecting the whole people, [could] be irrevocably fixed by decisions of the Supreme Court, the instant they are made in ordinary litigation between parties, in personal actions.' If that were to occur, said Lincoln, 'the people will have ceased to be their own rulers, having to that extent practically resigned the government into the hands of that eminent tribunal.'"*[19]

The Supreme Court made a terrible error in Roe v. Wade (as they did in the Dred Scott case). Those who try to defend it have to perform all kinds of verbal and political tricks. Those who work to overturn Roe v. Wade seek to change not only an immoral law, but seek to restore sanity to a nation whose values are based on political expediency and correctness, rather than truth and justice.

When the supreme Court holds power beyond what was ever envisioned, and when nine individuals make laws by finding penumbras in the Constitution emanating from wherever they choose, we the people, have lost control. The justices who voted for Roe made a terrible error when they ruled that a woman's convenience and lifestyle should supersede an unborn child's right to life. I believe that pride of intellect and a "fullness of self" have played a big part in continuing that erroneous judgment, a decision that has led to a cheapening of human life, escalated violence, physical and sexual abuse, and a general moral weakening of our government and our society.

---

[1] John Noonan, *A Private Choice*, The Free Press, McMillan Publishing, NY, 1979, p. 9.
[2] Marvin Olasky, *The Press and Abortion*, Lawrence Erblum Assoc., Hillsdale, N.J., 1988,

p. 117.
[3] From "A Freedom Fighter Packs for Washington," *Los Angeles Times*, March 8, 1993, View section, p.1.
[4] Ibid.
[5] Ibid.
[6] Editorial, the Los Angeles *Daily News*, July 12, 1993, p. 10.
[7] Ibid.
[8] Rabbi Daniel Lapin,, from a *Focus on the Family* radio broadcast, "Examining the Roots of Judeo Christian Values, Colorado Springs, Co. 1996.
[9] Robert P. Casey, "The Pro-life Principle Prevails: Dred Scott, Again," in *Crisis, A Journal of Lay Catholic Opinion*, p. 16.
[10] Robert P. Casey, "The Politics of Abortion," *The Human Life Review*, The Human Life Foundation, Inc., New York, N.Y. Summer 1992, p. 44.
[11] Ibid.
[12] Robert P. Casey, from a speech "The Pro-life Principle Prevails: Dred Scott, Again," in *Crisis, A Journal of Lay Catholic Opinion*, Brownstone Institute, Inc., Notre Dame, Ind., 1993, p. 17.
[13] Henry Hyde, in *For Every Idle Silence*, Servant Books, Ann Arbor, Michigan, 1985.
[14] Ibid., p 12.
[15] Ibid., pp. 12 & 13.
[16] Robert P. Casey, "The Pro-life Principle Prevails: Dred Scot, Again," in *Crisis, A Journal of Lay Catholic Opinion*, Brownstone Institute, Inc., Notre Dame, Ind., 1993 p.22.
[17] from Radio Broadcast, Live from L.A., *KKLA, FM*, June 4, 1993, Jack Kocienski, the host.
[18] John Noonan, *A Private Choice*, The Free Press, McMillan Publishing, NY, 1979, p. 8.
[19] Robert P. Casey,, "The Pro-life Principle Prevails: Dred Scot, Again," in *Crisis, A Journal of Lay Catholic Opinion*, Brownstone Institute, Inc., Notre Dame, Ind., 1993 p. 20.

## Abortion & The Medically Correct

"Each individual human life begins at the beginning, at fertilization, and is a continuum from that time until death. Our government has the right and duty to protect the lives of all living humans in this nation regardless of place of residence (living in or out of the womb), degree of perfection, age, sex, or degree of dependency. This protection should be guaranteed by our Constitution and be enforced through due process of law. A civilization will ultimately be judged by how it treats the smallest, the most dependent, the most innocent among its members. Did that nation cherish, protect, love and nourish them--or kill them?"[1]           Jack Willke

The medical profession has developed a new code of morals and ethics: whatever works. They starve newborn babies who are imperfect because their parents ask them to. They keep aborted babies alive for awhile in order to use them for research. And, they kill unborn babies, perfect or imperfect, when they are inconvenient or an embarrassment to their parents or grandparents.

One of the reasons abortion has proliferated in this country is because of the lack of courage on the part of doctors who know abortion is wrong, but don't want to "make waves" or destroy the "old boy" referral network, even though they don't do abortions themselves.

It is estimated that only twenty-five percent of the doctors in this country perform abortions (at one and a half million per year!) Where are the other seventy-five percent and why aren't they speaking out? Don't they see what has happened? Aren't they appalled that baby-killing is big business? Possibly they don't want to be politically- or medically-incorrect? Most likely they don't want to get out of their comfort zones.

Dr. Jack Willke, one of the founders of the National Right to Life Committee, works tirelessly to educate this nation about the humanity of the unborn and the legal and political issues that surround the debate about legal abortion. Others, like Doctors James McMahon and Martin Haskell specialize in late-term abortions, and look upon their sophisticated methods of killing as an art form.

Still others, have changed their minds about their abortion practices. Dr. Bernard Nathanson, one of the founders of the National Abortion Rights action League, changed his mind completely after performing tens of thousands of abortions. In his book, *Aborting America*,[2] Dr. Nathanson describes how he and several others planned strategies for selling abortion to the American people. Among their plans was the use of the statistic that thousands of women died every year from illegal abortions. He says that they knew that was a lie, but it was a useful number, and they had no hesitation in using it. In fact, the year before Roe v. Wade was decided, in 1972, only 39 deaths from illegal abortions were officially reported.

Dr. Nathanson now works full-time, trying to educate us about the humanity of the unborn child. His two movies, *Silent Scream* and *Eclipse of Reason*, have become classic films in the education of the humanity of the unborn child. Using ultrasound, the unborn are shown, in utero, moving away from the sharp edge of the abortionist's knife, trying to move away from the pain and certain death.

One of the euphemisms used extensively to assure women that abortions are not morally or ethically wrong is that the unborn child is only a "blob of tissue." It has served physicians and activists well. Too bad it isn't truly medically-correct. The truth of the development of unborn children who are destroyed by abortion is much more sophisticated, as described by Dr. Bart T. Heffernan in *Abortion and Social Justice*:[3]

*"...This embryonic heart, which begins as a simple tube, starts irregular pulsations at twenty-four days which, in about one week, smooth into a rhythmic contraction and expansion..."*[4]

*"...By the end of the twentieth day the foundation of the child's brain, spinal cord and entire nervous system will have been established. By the sixth week after conception this system will have developed so well that it is controlling movements of the baby's muscles, even though the woman may not be aware that she is pregnant."*[5]

It is somewhat customary, now, to perform an ultrasound before performing the abortion, especially if the woman is not sure of the exact date of her last period, or of the date she might have conceived. So, as I said before, the ultrasound screen is turned from her view. And, the facts quoted above about the development of her pre-born child are not divulged. She is told only that what is inside of her is a *"blob of tissue."*

The unborn child is not a blob of tissue, even at the sixth week (when the earliest, safe abortions are performed), but he or she becomes a blob of tissue after being sucked out of the womb by the powerful vacuum in early abortions, or cut up and scraped out in later procedures.

If an abortion is "just a medical procedure," why can't the truth be given to women who "very seriously" consider their "choices?"

Many doctors, who don't perform abortions, feel that they must refer not only long-time patients, but new, unknown callers, to some abortionist, somewhere. So they will have their assistants and receptionists tell women to go to the Eve Surgical Clinic or a similar abortion chain. Eve's specialty, performed by Dr. James McMahon, are late-term abortions. He was the subject of a *Los Angeles Times* article in 1990. In that article he said that late term abortions are his "passion."[6] According to Karen Tumulty, the reporter:

*"McMahon says that his conscience and his religious beliefs (he still attends Mass occasionally) have answered the basic questions that arise from later abortions. 'I've always been a classic liberal. I believe in freedom in its broadest sense,' says the doctor, whose office is decorated with photographs of his own two children. 'I frankly think the soul or personage comes in when the fetus is accepted by the mother.'"*[7]

You and I have our personage or soul affirmed only when our mothers accept us? I wish I could think of a comment on such bizarre thinking, but it boggles my mind. Tumulty comments further:

*"He has outfitted his surgical center with hidden, Israeli-made steel shutters that drop over his plate-glass windows at the flip of a*

*switch.*"[8]

It was interesting to note that most of the clinic doctors or directors who spoke to Karen when she was writing the article wanted their names or the names of their clinics to remain anonymous. If abortion is not a shameful or illegal procedure, then why the need for anonymity? Is there a subconscious shame?

I have often wondered how doctors can go in day after day to an office where they will repeatedly kill unborn children. I have wondered how they go home at night to a family or alone and wash their hands before dinner without being able to wash off the blood. Maybe they leave their hearts and souls on the doorstep so they can deal with what they do every day in the abortion clinic. Maybe the following passage from the book, *One Generation After*, by Elie Wiesel, offers some insight into how they handle the situation. Mr. Wiesel was writing about his thoughts as he entered Auschwitz as a prisoner.

> *"Think of your soul and you'll resist better. The soul is important and the enemy knows it; that's why he tries to corrupt it before destroying us. Do not let him. The soul counts for more than the body. If your soul maintains its strength, your body too will withstand the test. I tell you this because you have just arrived; you are still capable of listening. In a month it will be too late. In a month you will no longer know what having a soul could possibly mean."*[9]

Dr. Nathanson wrote in *Aborting America*:

> "I believe that an unexamined utilitarian ethos, and a corresponding 'situation ethic' have led us to this monstrous abortion situation. Instead of cherishing the individual human life, we are calculating the 'greatest good for the greatest number,' which translates into quality of life..."[10]

Dr. George Flesh, a Los Angeles obstetrician, who performed abortions as part of his practice, changed his mind several years ago. He published an article in the *Los Angeles Times* in 1991, telling why he no longer performs abortions. I met Dr. Flesh a few months later, after I had written a short article about him for our newsletter. He told me that since his *Times'* article was published, he had changed his mind about even referring a client for abortion. He said that now he will take extra time with a woman seeking an abortion, giving her complete information on the physical risks of abortion and information on the development of her unborn baby. From Dr. Flesh's original article:

> *"...a married couple came to me and requested an abortion. Because the patient's cervix was rigid, I was unable to dilate it to perform the procedure. I asked her to return in a week, when the cervix would be softer.*
> 
> *The couple returned and told me that they had changed their minds and wanted to 'keep the baby.' I delivered the baby seven months later. Years later, I played with little Jeffrey in the pool at the tennis club where his parents and I were members. He was happy and beautiful. I was horrified to think that only a technical obstacle had prevented me from terminating Jeffrey's potential life.*
> 
> *The connection between a 6-week old human embryo and a laughing child stopped being an abstraction for me. While hugging my sons each morning, I started to think of the vacuum aspirator that I would use two hours later. This was an emotional tension I could not tolerate."*[11]

Dr. Flesh has been an obstetrician-gynecologist for sixteen years. He was trained at UCLA Medical Center, and then was a resident at L. A. County Hospital. As a resident, the physicians were taught to do abortions. I asked if any of his colleagues had refused to do them. He said that only one out of the twelve residents he was with had not participated.

He said that he had been doing about one or two abortions per week at the time he began to question the morality of what he was doing. It had been a gradual shift in his thinking. He said that the decision to stop performing all abortions was made as he was praying in his synagogue on Yom Kippur. He said that at that moment of decision, he felt a lightness of spirit he hadn't experienced in a long time. Later that day, at a social gathering, (he had not even told his wife yet of this decision) he sensed a renewal and enthusiasm for his career and his personal life that he had not felt for some time.

After the article appeared, he received letters from all over the world, either supporting him or criticizing him about his public change of heart. He also received letters from irate patients, who said they would no longer come to him as a patient. His practice did suffer. Some did not write--they just cancelled appointments or found a new ob/gyn. He did receive, however, a few new patients who wanted a physician who did not perform abortions.

Some of his colleagues were astonished that he could make that decision and then write publicly about it. A woman obstetrician was especially vehement about his article. She was moved to write a letter to the *Los Angeles Times* in defense of abortion, in opposition to Dr. Flesh's article.

In her letter, she stated that because of fetal abnormalities alone, abortion should remain legal. How could he not do abortions for that reason? Even though in his article, Dr. Flesh had left open the option of abortion for fetal anomaly, she refused to acknowledge his concession to abortion for those reasons. In our most recent conversation, Dr. Flesh told me that by the end of 1991 he had changed his view of abortion in the case of birth defects, also, even though he had not thought that way originally. He said that he doesn't understand our society's overwhelming need for perfection. He now believes that all life should have a chance.

Handicapped people do live valuable lives. Chronically ill, wheel-chair bound, or retarded individuals can and do experience happiness. Besides, we are only guaranteed the right to the pursuit of happiness by our Constitution, not the state of happiness itself. There are so many diverse factors contributing to happiness that no one can really decide who is happy, or who will or won't be happy after they are born. Those who say that abortion is "for the child's sake" have got to be disingenuous or very confused. Dr. Fred Mecklenburg wrote in the book, *Abortion and Social Justice*:

*"It has been, of course, frequently pointed out that mentally and physically retarded citizens will never enjoy the delights of intellectual or physical achievement known to the normal person. This is true. However, by the same token, the normal person can never enjoy the intellectual excellence of the genius or the physical prowess of the athlete. And yet, this is hardly sufficient cause for considering the elimination of all but the genius and the athlete."*[12]

I counseled a woman once, who had been told at about five months into her pregnancy that her unborn child had hydrocephalus. She had two young daughters already, whom she had been involving in her pregnancy experience. Although they were not able to see the movements of the unborn baby yet, she would tell them when he was moving and place their hands on her stomach.

She came to me very distressed because the doctor was advising abortion as soon as possible, and her husband was also pressuring for the abortion. She said that she had already bonded with her child, as had her children. She knew that the short time that her child would most likely live would be heartbreaking, but at least she would have those memories of her son or daughter. And, carrying the baby to term, experiencing whatever would come would be natural, and she would not have to feel that she had participated in his or her early death by abortion. She was one of the strongest ladies I have ever met. I could only listen and try to understand her feelings.

She came in a second time with her husband so that she could explain herself better, and, maybe persuade him to see her viewpoint. She wanted him to see someone other than the doctor who was actively promoting the abortion. Her husband was polite, but he said the economic considerations, and the actual fact of the certain early death of the child made him think she should have the abortion. I didn't hear from them again. Sadly, I'm almost positive that she was eventually talked into the abortion.

In the case of spina bifida, often cited as a reason for abortion, the disease is not necessarily fatal, and victims can often live fairly normal lives. My son went to school with a young woman, who, though she had to have many surgeries because of her spina bifida, was a good student, a happy and accomplished

# Abortion & the Medically-Correct

individual. She is now in college, doing well.

The social pressures placed on pregnant women by physicians and others for abortions, even when there is no known medical reason for one are very intimidating. I heard from the grandmother of an aborted child a few days after the procedure. Her daughter was aborted even though she had told the doctor several times that her daughter was not a good candidate for an abortion, and the young woman had told the doctor the day before that she didn't really want one. She was, obviously, conflicted about her decision and was only there because of her boyfriend's pressure.

The doctor, however, did not listen. Instead, he promoted his own agenda regarding abortion for unmarried girls. He told the pregnant teen and her mother about his granddaughter. She had her own room and her own computer. He asked what *she, the pregnant teen,* thought she could do for her child after it is born. The pregnant girl had answered, "But, what about love and the care I will give my child?"

As she was being wheeled into the operating room the next day, she was crying and saying that she had changed her mind. When the nurse turned to the doctor and asked if they should stop, he said, "No," and continued with the procedure.

The grandmother and mother of that unborn baby both deeply regret the abortion. They want to take legal action against this doctor, but I'm willing to bet that the emotional involvement in such action will be so draining that the doctor's actions will probably never be publicly called into question. Several years ago a woman called me who had hired an attorney. She had nearly died in an abortion clinic because of negligence. She was married and had sought the abortion without the knowledge of her husband. After the abortion, as she lay in recovery, she was hemorrhaging and her blood pressure was dangerously low. The doctor kept saying that she would be all right. Finally, after the doctor left, the nurse said, "The hell with what the doctor said," and called for an ambulance to take the bleeding woman to a hospital.

Later that night, when the woman's husband had been called, another doctor said he didn't think he could save her--she was very near death. Her uterus had been perforated and she had lost too much blood. He had performed a complete hysterectomy. She miraculously survived, however, but deeply regretted the abortion, and was very angry about the doctor's negligence. When the attorney she had hired tried to find the nurse who had saved her life, he found that she no longer worked at that clinic. Whether she left on her own, or was conveniently let go I never did find out.

I have been told that doctors whose main business is abortion are not accepted in the medical community on a social level--that there is an avoidance of them, personally, and a neglect of discussions about their practice. But, abortionists support one another.

Recently, Dr. McMahon, who is "passionate" about abortion, testified in support of a Dr. Kinneally, who is the director of several abortion clinics, known as *Her* Medical Clinics. Dr. Kinneally was being investigated on wrongful death charges in several cases at his clinic. Later, during a court break, they discussed their late term abortion techniques and voiced admiration for one another on their expertise.

*"'There's a great deal of craft to this procedure,' says James McMahon, who employs two staff doctors. He doesn't allow doctors to work for him until they have performed at least 600. 'Frankly,' he added, I don't think I was any good at all until I had done 3,000 or 4,000.'"*[13]

Dr. McMahon is, most likely, a great admirer of Dr. Martin Haskell, who developed the D and X (dilation and extraction) method of abortion. Dr. Mc Mahon uses this particularly gruesome method for some of his mid- and late-term abortions.

The different types of abortion procedures need to be discussed, though it's always difficult to read the truth about abortion. I detail here each of six methods used and their descriptions. These are reprinted from a pamphlet, "Abortion: Some Medical Facts," published by the Life Education Fund.[14]

***Suction Aspiration.*** *Suction aspiration abortion (or menstrual extraction if done early in pregnancy) is used in 95% of induced abortions. A* powerful suction tube is inserted into the womb through the dilated cervix. This dismembers the body of the developing baby and tears the placenta from the uterus, sucking them into a container. These body parts are usually recognizable as arms, legs, head, etc. Great care must be used to prevent the uterus from being punctured during this procedure. Uterine hemorrhage and infection can easily result if any fetal or placental tissue is left behind in the uterus.

**Dilatation and Curettage.** *In this technique the cervix is dilated or stretched to permit insertion of a loop shaped steel knife in order to scrape the wall of the uterus. This cuts the baby's body into pieces and cuts the placenta from the uterine wall. Bleeding is sometimes considerable. This method is used primarily during the seventh to twelfth week of pregnancy and should not be confused with therapeutic D & C done with a blunt curette for reasons other than undesired pregnancy.*

**Dilatation and Evacuation (D&E)** *Used to remove a child from the womb who is as old as 18 weeks, this method is similar to the D & C. The difference is that a forceps is used to grasp part of the developing baby who already has calcified bones. The parts must be twisted and torn away, the placenta sliced away and bleeding is profuse.*

**Salt Poisoning:** *Otherwise known as "saline amniocentesis" or "salting out," this technique is used after 16 weeks of pregnancy, when enough fluid has accumulated in the amnionic fluid sac surrounding the baby. A needle is inserted through the mother's abdomen directly into the sac, and a solution of concentrated salt is injected into it. The baby breathes in, swallowing the salt and is thereby poisoned. After about an hour, the child dies, and the mother usually goes into labor approximately a day later, delivering a dead, burned and shriveled baby. This is the second most common method of inducing abortion. It is outlawed in Japan and other countries because of its inherent risks to the mother.*

**Prostaglandin Abortions:** *Prostaglandins are hormones which assist the birth process. Injecting concentrations of them into the amnionic sac induces violent labor and premature birth of a child usually too young to* *survive. Oftentimes salt or another toxin is first injected to assure that the baby will be delivered dead, since some babies have survived the trauma of prostaglandin birth at this stage, and have been delivered alive. This method is usually used during the second half of the pregnancy. A self-administered prostaglandin suppository or tampon is also being developed for first trimester abortion. Serious side effects and complications from prostaglandins use, including cardiac arrest, and rupture of the uterus, can be unpredictable and very severe.*

**Hysterotomy:** *Similar to the Caesarean Section, this method is generally used if the salt poisoning or prostaglandin methods fail. Sometimes babies are born alive during this procedure which raises questions as to how and when the infants are killed and by whom. Some infants who are attended to after a hysterotomy have been known to survive and were subsequently accepted by their natural mothers, or placed in adoptive homes. This method offers the highest risk to the health of the mother. The risk of mortality from hysterotomy is two times greater than risk from D & E.*

If abortion is ever fully accepted, will assisted suicide and euthanasia next become medically- and socially-correct?

When we took our daughter to the hospital to have her first baby, at three in the morning, she was given several documents to read and sign. Because her water had broken, and she was nervous, she asked me to read the document, entitled "Living Will." My daughter was being asked to sign, at 3:00 AM, in the beginning of her labor, a document that would have enabled the hospital to disconnect her from life support if there were complications and it was determined that her death would be imminent. She had her husband and her parents there with her to read this for her, but I thought about those who come into the hospital alone in an emergency, having just been in an accident, or in the midst of severe vomiting from food poisoning, or bleeding heavily from a miscarriage. Do they have this thing shoved at them or a friend or relative? Do they sign this frightening document?

Last November, Proposition 161 was narrowly defeated in California. A similar proposition had been narrowly defeated in the State of Washington earlier. The proposal would have made legal, assisted suicides. I read this proposed piece of legislation thoroughly. If it had become law, we all would be in jeopardy. With this law in place, assisted suicide and euthanasia could be implemented if a person had said more than once that he wished he could die.

Now, luckily, I have only experienced terrible pain (other than childbirth) a few times in my life, but I remember thinking a couple of times, when I had very painful headaches from a cold or a flu, "If only I could be put out of my misery!" In fact, I remember articulating that once or twice. What if I had been in the hospital, had signed the "Living Will" document, and what if, twice, someone had heard me? I would be a candidate for active euthanasia. However, according to Proposition 161, if I were to call the physician before he "did it" I could retract my death wish. That is, if his answering service could find him before his designated medical assistant had given me a lethal dose of something or other.

What will happen when this proposed legislation comes up again? Will we be indoctrinated sufficiently by that time? Will the subtle suggestion that old people should *die with dignity* and unburden their families be well-entrenched in our collective psyche?

Does being able to do a thing mean we need to do it? Doctors think that they hold the keys to life, that they can be gods if they want. We've taken the true God and His plan for nature out of procreation. We've fertilized a human ovum with a human sperm in a petri dish. Next, an artificial womb will be able to nurture the petri-dish embryos. No real humans needed for natural, sexual procreation. Will we eventually have the ability to make clones for individual tasks? Will there be a new age of slavery? I wonder if there will be a Dred Scott decision or an Emancipation Proclamation for cloned human beings! God help us. I hope I'm not around for all of this. Unfortunately, my grandchildren and my great grandchildren will be.

The health of the mother, both physiological and psychological, was used as the need for legal abortions before Roe v. Wade. That thinly disguised reason for therapeutic abortion used in California, Colorado, and other states at that time does not even need to be used today. Again, from Dr. Mecklenburg, in *Abortion and Social Justice*:

> *"In Colorado, 71.5% of all abortions are performed on psychiatric grounds (29), in Oregon, 97% (30), and in California, 90% (31). If we are to believe these figures (and there is little doubt as to their accuracy), then we must be willing to accept the fact that in these states serious mental illness is 15-20 times greater than physical illness in pregnant women (32), and that 25-50% of pregnant women are mentally ill. What in reality began as limited abortion in these states has now become (also in reality) abortion-on-demand, and this is primarily due to gross abuse of the mental health clause which obtains in each of these states."*[15]
>
> *"...Psychiatrists in these states and others have allowed themselves to be prostituted, misrepresenting social problems and personal inconvenience as 'grave impairments to mental health.'"*

But, even though a *mental health* excuse is really not needed today, I would like to discuss abortion for reasons of psychological well-being because that is still offered as rationalization for abortion. Dr. Fred Mecklenburg continued:

> *"Threat to the Mental Health of the Mother. There are no known psychiatric diseases which can be cured by abortion. In addition, there are none which can be predictably improved by abortion. Noyes and Kolbe's standard textbook of psychiatry, used in most medical schools in the United States, states that 'experience does not show that pregnancy and the birth of the child influence adversely the course of schizophrenia, manic depressive illness or the majority of psychoneuroses.*[16]
>
> *"Paradoxically, the very women for whom legal abortion may seem most justifiable are also the ones for whom the risk is highest for post-abortion psychic insufficiency.*
>
> *"It should be pointed out that suicide in the pregnant woman is extremely rare. In fact, it is about 1/6 the rate seen in nonpregnant women of the same age..."*[17]
>
> *"...Lindberg, in Sweden, while studying 304 patients whose request for therapeutic abortion had been refused, observed that not one*

*actually committed suicide; although 62 indicated they would if their request was refused.*"[18]

I submit that those who are truly mentally disturbed are most likely not to seek an abortion. As an example, one of our clients, who was obviously an emotionally disturbed woman was also very nice. I liked Jan and felt sorry for her. She was very distressed about her pregnancy, and said that she was getting a lot of pressure to abort her unborn child. She desperately wanted to have the baby.

I offered to get her professional psychiatric help, but Jan told me that she already had a psychiatrist, and that she had been on medications for her mental problems, but she didn't want to take them during this time. She had had two abortions previously. She had been married at one time, but lost her two young children to the custody of their father. After counseling her several times, I suggested that she consider adoption. This nearly destroyed our fragile relationship. She had *lost* too many children already, she said. She wanted to raise this child herself. All of our counselors who received calls from her throughout her pregnancy worked with her by simply listening, and being there for her.

Jan called, finally, from the hospital, to tell us she had had a daughter. Medical personnel must have judged that she was competent to keep the baby, because after the birth she took the baby home, went back on her medications, and appeared to be doing well.

I wish I could say that that was the end of the story and that it was a happy ending, but not exactly. She contacted me about six weeks later, saying that she was very upset; she had taken the baby into the local hospital twice that week because "she wasn't breathing right" and she had a fever. She said that at that moment she wasn't breathing right again, and maybe Jan had eaten something bad and when the baby nursed she got the "bad stuff."

She had never given me her phone number or address before. She was always sure we would try to take her baby away from her. But, when she needed help in this situation, she gave me her address and allowed me to come to her apartment. I drove over, hoping that there wouldn't really be an emergency. The baby seemed listless, and a little warm. Jan's apartment was not neat, but seemed to be clean. The baby's bed was a bassinet that had been detached from its legs. It was sitting on the floor.

I couldn't really decide if there was a medical emergency or not, but Jan was close to hysteria. I decided to call the paramedics. I hoped they would make the judgment about the baby's health and about the possible need to take some further action. Eventually, when I explained to the paramedics about Jan's history and my worry about her judgment and competence, the police were called, and Jan and the baby were driven to the hospital in their van.

Now, I know there are those who would say that she should never have had the baby, that she might have harmed the child or worse. And, I say that at least the baby was given life, given a chance. I'm sorry for Jan and her anguish, but sometimes tough choices need to be made for everyone. A week after I went with Jan and her daughter to the hospital, I went over to the apartment to bring a little dress for the baby. She told me then that Children's Services had placed the baby in a foster home, pending a court hearing. I had such mixed emotions about my involvement. Certainly the welfare of the child was paramount, but the loss that Jan felt again was so sad. At least her daughter had a chance. No one would have benefited--not Jan, her daughter, or adoptive parents if she had had the abortion.

What about pregnant women whose physical life is threatened by a pregnancy? Dr. Mecklenburg spoke about this in the same article quoted above:

*"A small number of pregnant patients with severe renal disease and decompensating renal function seem truly threatened by pregnancy. Even in this instance, however, heroic measures such as the use of a dialysis unit may see these women through severe life-threatening episodes."*[9]

I used to work for a physician who was in charge of the Nephrology Division of the Department of Medicine at UCLA. At that time, the early days of organ transplantation, many of the renal patients did not experience successful transplants--many kidneys were rejected. If the first transplanted kidney didn't take, another donor might be looked for and found. If a second transplant did not work, the patient might have to be kept alive with continuing hemodialysis.

I got to know some of the patients very well. One of them, whom I especially liked, was a 20-year old woman, Caren, who was given a cadaver transplant. She did surprisingly well and her prognosis was very good.

Shortly afterwards, she met and married a young man. Probably on the honeymoon, she became pregnant. Caren was seen by several doctors in the renal unit, and was advised to get an immediate abortion, as a pregnancy might seriously affect her delicate health. She had the abortion, without much time for deliberation.

By this time, I was a Mom myself, no longer working, but Caren, who lived near me, came to tell me about what had happened. She also told me that she regretted the abortion, and that she was again pregnant (about two months after the abortion). She said she was determined to go through with it, have a tubal ligation, and possibly, eventually, adopt a child to complete their family. And that is just what she did! She had a little girl, adopted another, and eventually went back to work.

In all fairness to women with serious health concerns, I don't know if I would have been as brave as Caren. I might have had the abortion. I just don't know. I had seen and gotten to know enough renal patients who died from less serious threats to their lives. I knew how precarious a kidney transplant patient's health was. Caren took the chance, and beat the odds. I applaud her for her courage. I've lost touch with her in the last few years, but if she ever chances to read this, I hope she knows how much I admire her. And, I hope her daughters know the full story of her illness and pregnancies.

How do doctors feel about physicians who regularly perform abortions? Doctors can always wash their hands of any responsibility for their colleagues' actions. They can always say, "I would never do abortions, but Dr. Mc Mahan has a right to do them, if he so chooses." They can always say that the patient has her right to choose and, therefore, I must refer her to another doctor. But, why can't they say to the patient that an abortion really is not an answer to your problem. Why not, "Please carefully consider what you are doing. There are risks to you, and you are carrying your own child inside of you?" Physicians used to take the Hippocratic Oath which includes the phrase, "I will do no harm." Why is it no longer medically-correct? What has changed?

Physicians who believe in the sanctity of human life should be in the forefront of the fight against abortion, rather than standing back. They should take a chance like Dr. Flesh did, by going public with their philosophy or they should, at least, face abortion and what it is truly doing to women, and then present those facts to their patients. It's true they will have to get out of their *comfort zones*, but possibly the sense of peace that they will experience in their hearts and minds will more than compensate for their initial discomfort.

---

[1] Jack Willke, M.D., from "When does Human Life Begin?" in *Life Cycle* pamphlet, #108 (10/81), published by WCCL Education Fund, Inc., Milwaukee, Wis., 1981.
[2] Bernard Nathanson, M.D., *Aborting America*, Doubleday and Co., Garden City, N.Y., 1979, p. 251.
[3] Bart T. Heffernan, from a chapter, "The Early Biography of Every Man," in *Abortion and Social Justice*, Sun Life, Thaxton, Virginia, 1980.
[4] Ibid., p. 5.
[5] Ibid.
[6] Karen Tumulty, "The Abortions of Last Resort," *Los Angeles Times Magazine*, 1/7/90, p. 10.
[7] Ibid.
[8] Ibid., p. 12.
[9] Elie Wiesel, *One Generation After*, trans. by Lily Edelman and the author (New York: Random House, 1970), pp 79-80.
[10] Bernard Nathanson, M.D., *Aborting America*, Doubleday & Co., Garden City, N.Y., 1979, p. 251.

[11] George Flesh, M.D., "Why I No Longer Do Abortions," *Los Angeles Times*, 9/12/91, Op-Ed section.

[12] Fred E. Mecklenburg, M.D., from "The Indications for Induced Abortion: A Physician's Perspective," in *Abortion and Social Justice*, Sun Life, Thaxton, Virginia, 1980, p. 44.
[13] Karen Tumulty, "The Abortions of Last Resort," *Los Angeles Times Magazine*, 1/7/90, p. 35.
[14] from the Pamphlet, entitled, "Abortion: Some Medical Facts," published by the National Right To Life Education Fund, 1984, 1988, 1989, 1991.
[15] Fred E Mecklenburg, M.D., from a chapter, "The Indications for Induced Abortion: A Physician's Perspective," in *Abortion and Social Justice*, Sun Life, Thaxton, Virginia, 1980, p. 41.
[16] Ibid., p. 39.
[17] Ibid., p. 40.
[18] Ibid.
[19] Ibid., p. 38.

# Used Women: Abortion & Big Business

"It is heartening to realize that now, after January, 1973, more than half of the 3.8 billion people of the world reside in political jurisdictions where abortion is permitted not only for medical but for sociological reasons as well. Liberalization of abortion is a rapidly progressing socio-legal phenomenon; it can not and will not be stopped until it is global in application."[1]

_____Alan F. Guttmacher

This foreword by Alan F. Guttmacher for the book, *Abortion: A Woman's Guide*, was a prophecy and a dream (of his and Planned Parenthood's) that have, for the most part, come true. But, the staggering emotional and physical damage to millions of women, worldwide, is pandemic. I have met many of the damaged ones.

It has been estimated that the abortion industry makes about $500 million dollars a year. If you think about it, this is money made at the cost of over one and a half million unborn children's lives. The damage to their mothers, both psychologically and physiologically is uncountable. The good news for doctors is that a woman can be aborted more than once. The bad news is women never truly benefit from the experience. They are only used.

In an abortion, the cervix, (which is meant to open gradually, near the time of natural delivery of a woman's baby) is wrenched open. This forced stretching destroys the strength and elasticity of the cervix, which often leads to multiple miscarriages in subsequent pregnancies. These might well be pregnancies that are now intended and welcomed, but, because of the cervical damage, are naturally aborted at about twelve weeks. The vacuuming process used in early abortions with a vacuum aspirator imposes further damage. The uterus was never meant to be invaded by a machine that can nick and scratch its delicate lining. If scarring occurs near the opening of the fallopian tubes, a fertilized ovum may be too large to fit and, thus, cannot pass through into the uterus. If the fetus begins to develop in the tube, a dangerous ectopic pregnancy can occur. Indeed, the occurrence of ectopic pregnancies has "strangely" multiplied in the two decades since legalized abortion.

The latest development in abortions, dilation and extraction, (D & X) is designed for fetal-parts' harvesting to be used for experimentation and transplantation, and for ease of

# Used Women: Abortion & Big Business

removal of the later-term unborn child, who is usually too large for the unsoftened cervix. To begin treating unborn babies as a commodity, a resource for research and transplantation of body parts into *useful* "products of conception" is a frightening slip on the slippery slope. To use women for this type of supposedly humanitarian purpose is the beginning of the total disintegration of any societal regard or protection for human life.

There are many popular arguments used for abortion, especially for those unborn babies whose birth would be abhorrent to individuals or society in general. Rape is one of the most overused examples of a need for legal abortion.

Very early one morning, I was asked the big question about one of those cases: "What about a woman who has been raped? Shouldn't she be able to get an abortion?" A small radio station somewhere in Northern California called our hotline on a sleepy Sunday morning. The host wanted to interview someone about an abortion decision the Supreme Court had handed down the day before, the Webster decision, which let stand some previously enacted Missouri laws against abortion. The show's host was gracious enough to tell me before I went on, live, that he wasn't going to be so nice at the time of broadcast. I agreed to the interview, anyway--I think I was still half asleep.

His first question was the other biggie: "Is abortion murder?" I replied that it certainly was a question of taking human life, but every homicide must be determined in the courts if it is an act of murder or not. That crime, in each individual case, is decided by a prosecutor, a jury and a judge.

I'm not even sure I had ever answered that question in that manner before, but it seemed passable, considering the time I had been given to think and speak at that early hour. I was not prepared for the next question, however.

"Have you seen the movie, *The Accused*?" I knew the movie was based on the true story of a woman who was gang-raped in a revolting way in a bar, on a pool table, somewhere on the East Coast. I said I had not seen the movie, but I was aware of the subject matter. The radio show host then asked, "Don't you think that if she had gotten pregnant from that brutal rape she should have had an abortion? Not even being able to determine the father of the child?"

I replied that an abortion is another act of violence. She had been treated in a despicable, disgusting way, but another act of violence, an abortion, would do nothing but establish in the victim's mind that she is dirty, a piece of trash, a problem to be disposed of. For her to be treated as a pariah by family, friends, and a doctor who all pressure her into an abortion, confirms, in her mind, that she has been defiled or is guilty. Both experiences are violent, both have a negative, traumatic ending. In both cases she is a victim.

Victims of rape who became pregnant were the subject of a study done by Dr. Sandra Mahkorn, which was published in a book, *Psychological Aspects of Abortion*.[2] Dr. Mahkorn is a rape counselor, who, in 1979, identified 37 pregnant rape victims who had been treated by a social welfare agency. Twenty-eight of the thirty-seven women gave birth. Seventeen chose adoption, three raised the child themselves, and the whereabouts of the other eight women could not be determined.

Several of the women interviewed stated that they felt an abortion would have been another act of violence. Some felt that there was an intrinsic value in the child they carried to term--somehow there was a hidden purpose for this "unwanted baby."

Certainly, subconsciously, (if not consciously) the victim of rape feels that if she can get through the pregnancy she will have been able to overcome the violation of her body and the lingering traumatic effects. By giving life to the child, she is empowered and establishes herself as better than the rapist, a fact that subliminally, at first, she is not sure of. They are courageous women, those who choose not to become a victim a second time.

I counseled a young woman by phone, who, even though she was only thirteen, called me on her own. Her family had said that her pregnancy was her problem. She told me that she had just found out she was pregnant. She was about sixteen weeks into the pregnancy. She had been raped on her way home from school by a stranger. She hadn't even told anyone about the rape, until she found out she was pregnant.

I put her in touch with two public health nurses who got her immediate medical care. I also asked for help from a church group called Loving Decisions, who befriended her and helped her with all of her practical needs. They drove her to doctor's appointments, got maternity clothes for her--whatever help they could give.

I never met Angie, but I did speak to her after the baby was born and given to adoptive parents. She said that it had been hard to give up the baby, even under the circumstances of the rape and her young age. I've never forgotten Angie and her story. I hope she has healed from that terrible crime. I'm glad there were so many to help her when she needed support.

Women who are raped are used as objects to satisfy some

inner rage. It's not a loving act, nor is it even a sexy act. Likewise, women who are used as objects in the abortion industry are a commodity, a human product used to satisfy a doctor's greed. Their bodies are great little moneymakers, and with a little luck for the abortionist, the same woman can be aborted over and over again. Lee Ezell was a rape victim who became pregnant from the assault. She now regularly speaks out about her experience. She wrote a book, *The Missing Piece*,[iii] about her life before and after this crime. I first read an article Lee had written about rape and pregnancy in the *Los Angeles Times*. And, I heard Lee speak about her experience in April of 1993. This is a bit of her story.

In June of 1962, Lee, her sister, and her mother, moved to San Francisco, in an attempt to escape a lifetime of abuse by Lee's father, who was an alcoholic. Lee found a job with a small sailboat company. One of the salesmen, who only came occasionally into the office, invited her and a couple of her new friends to join him at his house to have pizza and watch television that evening. Lee followed him over in her car, while the other young women went to buy the pizza. Almost as soon as she arrived, the man assaulted and raped her. She got out of the house as soon as he was through with her. She was shaken and sick inside, but able to hide what had happened, or so she thought. Her plan was to go on with her life without telling anyone. After all, her mother and sisters were starting a new life. She was only eighteen, and had been a virgin.

When she found out that she was pregnant, and finally told her family, her mother decided that she should move out. Lee, distraught, did not try to explain. She moved to Southern California, got a new job, and began living with a married couple she met at church. She soon became confident enough of their friendship that she told them the truth about her rape and pregnancy. They lovingly supported her in her desire not to have an abortion, but to give birth to the child, and to put her own and the child's future in God's hands.

Lee had a little girl, who was adopted by a couple, who soon afterward moved to the Midwest. She lost touch with them.

When Lee finally met the man she was to marry she told him what had happened to her. Would he be able to accept her? He was a recent widower with two daughters. Would she be able to accept his girls as her own, and could they accept her? He also told Lee that he could not have any more children. Some tough decisions had to be made by all. Lee's only natural child might possibly be the one she had conceived from the rape and given to adoptive parents. After much consideration and prayer, she decided that she could love and care for these young girls who had tragically lost their own mother, and they would be her daughters.

After many years of marriage, Lee answered a very unexpected telephone call one day. The good friends she had lived with when she was pregnant had received a call and a letter from a girl named Julie, who said she was Lee's daughter. She said she wanted to find her mother. Julie was married and had just had a baby a few months earlier. She had been working with adoption search groups to try to find her birth mother. After several years, it looked like she had succeeded.

Lee gave the okay for her daughter to get in touch with her, and they finally met. Her "missing piece," Julie, was glad to be alive, and Lee was glad that she had made a positive decision twenty years earlier, instead of the negative abortion decision. She now had three daughters and a granddaughter!

Some women who have not been raped, but have had abortions that they regret, will also speak out. One of our speakers tells the dramatic story of her abortion. Before her appointment, she was repeatedly told not to wear pants for the procedure. She didn't question; she just followed doctor's orders. But she did wonder once or twice what difference it would make if she didn't wear a skirt or a dress.

She soon found out, and the straightforward, narrative style she uses when she describes her abortion experience is very powerful. They showed her into the room, laid her on the table, and told her to lift her skirt. "Whoosh! I was out of there in ten minutes. No medical history, no blood pressure even taken. I was next in line, and there were others out there on the assembly line who couldn't wait."

The time that was saved by her not having to change into a surgical gown or removing slacks or jeans would enable the abortionist to do more procedures that day, and thus more money would be made! Women are ushered into abortion clinics; they are told to lift their skirts; their babies are sucked out of their bodies; they are told to wait a half-hour or so in a recovery area, and then they are sent on their way, usually crying or in a state of shock.

Another demonstration of the assembly-line mentality that dominates in the abortion clinics is illustrated by a recent incident and death in Santa Ana, California.

*"The owner of a family-planning clinic has been arrested on suspicion of murder after a pregnant patient died under suspicious*

*circumstances...*"[4]

Not only did Angela Sanchez die at the Clinica Femenina de la Comunidad, but personnel at the clinic tried to hide the fact of her death from her children, who were waiting for her.

" *'We waited and waited and my mother didn't come out,'* Maria Sanchez said. *'One of the ladies told me that my mother said it was OK for me to drive my mother's car home. But I said, 'I can't drive. I'm only 12' I knew my mother wouldn't have said that.'*"[5]

"*About 1 PM., Hanna's (clinic owner) assistant came out and offered to take the two children to lunch,* Maria Sanchez said. *When they returned, Angela Sanchez's car was gone and Maria Sanchez said the assistant told her her mother had left to go to another clinic.*"[6]

Later, Maria's uncle, trying to find Angela, drove back to the clinic with Maria.

" *'I ran around to the passenger side and I saw my mother lying on the ground.'* Maria Sanchez said. *'I asked the two women from the clinic, 'What happened to my mother?' They said, 'She's dead.'*"[7]

This case was well reported by the Spanish speaking newspapers and news shows, but was almost totally ignored by the major media.

I attended a trial in El Monte where a *clinic trespasser*, Father Peter Irving, was being tried for blocking access to a particular clinic that regularly aborted Hispanic women. The Director of the clinic and the owner/physician were both testifying on this particular date. His clientele, the owner told the Court, were basically Hispanic women, who spoke little or no English. When asked about the care given before, during, and after the abortions, and how information was given to or obtained from their patients, it became clear that no one in the clinic spoke Spanish. The women to be aborted were ushered in, placed on the table, and the procedure was performed. If the women had a health problem that needed to be dealt with, or if they had questions concerning the abortion procedure, no one was able to help them.

Father Irving was on trial, not the clinic owner or director. The priest had committed a misdemeanor crime, trespass, and must be brought to justice. But, the negligent procedures followed in this and other clinics apparently is within the law or ignored.

Is abortion a safe, easy answer to a difficult problem? If it is, then why are there so many young women who come back to us shortly after an abortion desperately trying to get pregnant again to make up for the child that was lost? Or why do women come to us years later asking for help with their grief and despair over the baby they had aborted?

We are now seeing young women who have grown up with legalized abortion. They see that it is sanctioned by the government, their parents, their peers, and even some of their churches. These young women have friends who have had abortions who will tell them that it is the easy way out. They aren't told that abortion only solves their immediate problem. They don't know that they will never be the same again.

I had a call one day from a woman named Sarah, who had had an abortion five days earlier at a clinic. She had immediate reactions of grief and guilt. She kept repeating to me that no one had told her what it would be like. When she called the clinic where she had been aborted, they said that they couldn't help her. At the end of our conversation she said she was going to try to get pregnant again very soon because she knew that was the only thing that would help her with her heartache. Sarah was married. I often wonder if the marriage survived the abortion experience.

Single women who have been victims of abortion almost never continue the relationship with the father of the child. They feel a sense of abandonment, a feeling that they had had to deal with the pregnancy and abortion completely on their own. Sometimes the split comes when their boyfriends are against the abortion, themselves. In both cases, the emotions involved are too devastating to continue as lovers or even as friends. Many women are not able to conceive or carry subsequent pregnancies to term. Their grief and despair is doubly painful.

I spoke to a woman recently who has had four abortions, one miscarriage, and was considering another abortion. Lynne cried frequently because one of her babies had been aborted at twenty-two weeks. She has been living a dysfunctional life, and has used drugs frequently. Her abortions obviously didn't liberate her. Her circumstances (not holding a job for any length of time, going from one relationship to another without marriage or commitment, and use of drugs) are typical of women who have had one or more abortions. If Lynne had not had the first abortion she might have gone on to live a much more stable, reasonably happy life. She might have found her own self-worth and been able to say no to relationships with men who consistently used her for their own purposes.

Many women come to us for almost-monthly pregnancy tests. They are trying, subconsciously, to get pregnant to make up for a recent or past abortion. I think Stacey was one of the few who consciously understood that that was her objective.

She sought help for her emotional pain only two months after the procedure. She was one of the "lucky" ones who faced the truth that she had made a terrible mistake right away. She wanted to deal with her pain by getting pregnant again. The irony of her situation was that she had broken up with her boyfriend. Her financial circumstances were no different than they had been, and her rocky relationship with her mother had not changed. She was back to square one, with the same negatives in her life that led to her abortion. Only now she was trying to get pregnant deliberately!

Her story, though the pain is uniquely hers, is typical of many abortion experiences. It is very powerful, as she tells it:

*"In January 1991 I had an abortion. At the time, I was living at home, going to school and working. The guy I was with was a loser. He had no job and he was an alcoholic and drug addict. When I found out I was pregnant I was in shock. Although we hadn't been using birth control, I still couldn't believe it really happened.*

*"I knew if I had the baby I wouldn't want to give it up. And single motherhood was not something I was sure I was prepared for. When I told my mother I was pregnant, she told me an abortion was a good idea. All my friends advised me to get an abortion as well. My mother took me to the Family Planning Associates Clinic. I had to sign something that stated that I consented to the abortion and was not coerced into it. I was laid on a table with my legs in stirrups and the table was raised. Although I couldn't see what was going on, I heard and felt what he was doing. I remember my legs were shaking violently throughout the procedure. I was also crying hysterically. All I could think to myself was they are killing my baby. There will be no more baby. My unborn child was cut up, scraped and suctioned out of me. During the entire procedure, no one said anything to me.*

*"I never received any counseling prior to the procedure. There was no one to talk to about what was going to happen. Everyone was so cold. They didn't want to talk to you about anything because they were scared some women might change their mind. They didn't care that they*

were making money off of murdering unborn babies. They are baby killers. They only seemed interested in moving the women in and out as quickly as possible. Abortion is big business.

"I was so traumatized after having the abortion. I couldn't believe how much it affected me. I couldn't stop thinking about what I had done. Even counseling didn't make me feel better. The only thing that finally made me feel better was when I got pregnant in July 1991, and gave birth on April 20, 1992 to an 8 lb., 13 oz. beautiful, healthy baby girl. I am so thankful I have her."[8]

Stacey kept in touch with us, and when I asked her to put her feelings down on paper, after the birth of her daughter, she wrote the letter above. I then asked if I could publish it, as it was a very powerful story, and had so much of everywoman's story in it. She graciously allowed us to use her letter.

If you multiply Stacey's story by about four thousand, you might have a picture of what is going on all over our country, every day. Our hope is that Stacey will eventually find peace of mind. She has told me that she knows God has forgiven her, but that she is finding it hard to forgive herself. Our hope is that one day she will be completely healed from her abortion experience.

The Family Planning Associates Clinic that she talked about is one of a chain of clinics in Southern California. Dr. Edward Allred is the owner. Some of his clinics are open seven days a week. They outdo Planned Parenthood (the largest abortion provider in the country) in sheer numbers of abortions in this area. Allred owns several racetracks.

Who else, besides the doctor, benefits from abortion? Almost always, pregnant, single women are left "holding the bag." The minute some liberated man is told by a liberated woman that she is pregnant, he tells her either that "it's her decision," or that she must have an abortion because he's not ready to be a father. Some of these *not-ready-to-be's* are 29 or older.

Many women tell a story of only a short relationship of two or three months. They had become sexually involved immediately, and then are faced with an unplanned pregnancy. They don't even have a basis for a long-term relationship, let alone for marriage and a family. Or a woman tells a story of a long, committed relationship (possibly they have been living together or have talked about marriage in the future) and then the baby comes into the picture. The picture almost always changes dramatically, and the 29- or 39-year old man suddenly gets morning (and afternoon and evening) sickness. In most of these cases, the father of the child is "outta there." He sometimes leaves soon after he finds out about the pregnancy or he threatens to leave if she doesn't have the abortion. Many women submit to an abortion because of this pressure.

This, of course, is not true in all cases. But, even when he says he will be there for her, to support her, this does not usually mean financial or practical support. In fact, it usually just means that he will hang around as long as it's comfortable for him to do so, and the decision (responsibility) is entirely up to her.

In the last thirty years or so, women have not insisted on marriage. They bought the feminist line that freedom comes with sexual liberation. "If I can sleep with Lance or John, move in with him possibly, then I will be truly free. I will have what men have had all these years with the old double standard-- a free sexual lifestyle!"

If that was their thinking, and it seems to have been, they bought themselves a lie, and the consequences have been powerful and devastating to themselves, to the family, and to our nation! Women have been deceived and used, and they have pursued the lie with a strange eagerness. Why has the proliferation of pornography, the increase of sexual assault and physical abuse increased with liberation? Certainly, ideally, all of these terrible things should decrease with equality for women. Women may think they have gained something when they enter into sexual relationships and live together without marriage. But, in reality, they are more used.

Women are not freed by making the decision to have an abortion. They are enslaved. Rather than a new beginning, the fresh start, the solution that they seek from an abortion, is the beginning of a lifetime of traumatic, psychological damage that they have little control over. They are faced with the mental anguish of regret, guilt, and grief. And, often they experience feelings of abandonment by those people who should have supported them in order to continue the pregnancy, rather than encouraging their abortion decision. How often I have heard, "My boyfriend supports me in whatever I decide." She thinks he is being very brave and considerate. I think he is washing his hands of any responsibility, either way. He is in a win-win situation.

Forty percent of women who have one abortion will have two or more.[9] It took me a long time and many hundreds of counseling sessions to figure out why they had the second (or more) abortions. What eventually became clear is that the second abortion strengthens, validates, and supports the first one. She tells herself, with a second abortion, that the first one was the right thing to do, so: "Here I am, pregnant again. The abortion I had three months ago helped me and was the only thing I could do then, so it will be my choice this time, too."

The third and subsequent abortions are a real mystery to me. Possibly, a woman can become so blind to the life she is living, so out of control, that she continues the casual sex and abortion cycle, much as alcoholics or drug abusers continue with their addictions. A good friend of mine, Leane, said that her four abortions just became a way of life for her, a birth control method.

Leane was a nurse, a very competent one. She began working for an abortionist sometime after her first two abortions. He performed the other two procedures for her. She regrets every one of them, and has since married. She's gotten her life together, but she didn't do it alone. Her faith in God is very strong.

Leane currently leads a post-abortion support group and a pregnant singles group. She is employed as a prenatal nurse at a county clinic. When we first met she told me that she probably would never be able to get pregnant because she had so much scar tissue from the multiple abortions. However, she has remarkably just found out she's pregnant at age 41! She is one of the few aborted women I have met who has been truly healed. My prayer is that this pregnancy will produce the child she has longed for.

It would be great if her healing and wholeness could be the happy ending for all women who have been victims of abortion, but unfortunately it isn't. Usually, the only winners are the men who walk away from the problem and the abortionists who make their fortunes in the abortion industry. The losers are the women who are abandoned and the babies who are killed. In the abortion experience there are always two victims. One, of course, is the baby who is given no choice. The other is the aborted woman. It's true that she is not legally forced into this decision. She <u>does</u> have a *choice*. But much too often the subtle (and sometimes not so subtle) pressures from her parents, her boyfriend, her peers, or even her doctor are so overwhelming that she feels she has no alternative. If this is what liberation for women is all about, then we'd better find another way.

---

[1] Alan Guttmacher, , *Abortion: A Woman's Guide*, Planned Parenthood of New York City, Inc., Abelard-Schuman Ltd., 257 Park Ave., South, NewYork, NY, 10010, p. xii.

[2] Sandra Mahkorn, "Pregnancy and Sexual Assault," in *The Psychological Aspects of Abortion*, ed. Mall and Watts (1979) pp. 53-72.

[3] Ezell, Lee, *The Missing Piece*, Servant Publications, Ann Arbor, Mich., 1992.

[4] *Orange County Register*, Friday, January 22, 1993, Section B1, p. 1.

[5] Ibid., p. 3.

[6] Ibid.

[7] Ibid.

[8] from a letter written by Stacey (pseudonym) for publication and use by the Pregnancy Counseling Clinic, Mission Hills, Ca. 1992.

[9] *Just the Facts* brochure, published by Dayton Right to Life Society, 1990, Dayton, Ohio, 513/461-3625.

## *Liberated Women*

"The real change was women's new ability to regulate their fertility without danger or fear--the new freedom, that in turn had contributed to dramatic changes not in the abortion rate, but in female sexual behavior and attitudes. Having secured first the mass availability of contraceptive devices and then the option of medically sound abortions, women were at last at liberty to have sex, like men, on their own terms. As a result, in the half century after birth control was legalized, women doubled their rates of pre-marital sexual activity, nearly converging with men's by the end of the seventies."
_____Susan Faludi[1]

Faludi portrays feminism and the sexual revolution as positive and honorable. But, in her book, *Backlash*,[2] she is angry because she feels that these "liberties" are being eroded. She is angry because the sisterhood is standing back and allowing conventional ideas to stand. I see her, in this book, as the captain, on the bow of a sinking ship, calling back all of the deserting rats.

Some of the history of the women's liberation movement was described by Carole A. Wilk in her book, *Career Women and Childbearing*. In the following paragraph, she presents the societal backdrop and changes that contributed to the movement:

*"Our subjects' development during high school was powerfully influenced by the Vietnam crisis. Many of these fast-track kids became the Vietnam flower children. Whether they participated in active protest or not, dissent against the established system was validated. The loss of faith in authority and the loss of confidence in the legitimacy of traditional systems of restraint spilled over from the political/military domain (Watergate and Vietnam), to the personal/sexual/moral spheres. It became the rule, legitimate and expected, to challenge tradition. Frequently, the most familiar traditions, those closest and best-known, were attacked first. Thus, parents' roles, values, behaviors, relationships and life styles became a prime target. Our subjects looked critically at their parents: many felt a need to be different, especially a need to be different from mother. This challenge to tradition coincided with the growing power of the women's movement. The struggle to change the traditional secondary position of women, to formulate a new definition of*

# Liberated Women

*the feminine role, to allow women to develop according to unique, individual timetables, rather than to a prior set of social expectations, developed into a dominant social movement.*"[3]

Helen Gurley Brown took advantage of all of these changes in the sixties when she wrote her famous book, *Sex and the Single Girl*.[4] The only reason it was such a big seller and an important promotion of the sexual revolution was because she had the audacity to say *what* she did *when* she did. She claimed her liberation and promoted the same for her female readers by presenting her detailed plans for attracting, enjoying, and using men, without commitment--just as men had always treated women. She was the original, on-record, playgirl, I guess. She advocated multiple sexual partners. Even having two sexual relationships simultaneously could be a good thing! She told her readers how to decorate their apartments and give a chic dinner for two. She launched her career on this little masterpiece, and, to this day, remains the Editor of *Cosmopolitan Magazine*. Her use of women and their provocative, almost-bared breasts are the subject of every cover. She knows what sells. Never mind the fact that she is exploiting women for her marketing purposes.

How truly liberated have women become because of their increased sexual activity and their casual relationships, preferring to live together with men, rather than marrying and establishing a family? How liberating is their easy access to contraception and abortion?

The lie that proliferates among those who favor abortion is that the emotional reactions to, and the impact of, an abortion are not greater than the effects of childbirth.

Colmin McCarthy quoted Dr. Julius Fogel in his Commentary in the *St. Paul Sunday Pioneer Press*. Fogel is a psychiatrist-obstetrician, who performs abortion, but faces honestly the effects on the women he aborts:

*"'Abortion is an impassioned subject...Psychologically and emotionally we are only beginning to learn something of its effects on the women involved. I think every woman--whatever her age, her background or sexuality--has a trauma at destroying a pregnancy. A level of humanness is touched. This is a part of her own life. She destroys a pregnancy; she is destroying herself. There is no way it can be innocuous. One is dealing with the life force. It is totally beside the point*

*whether or not you think life is there. You cannot deny that something is being created and that this creation is physically happening.*'"⁵

There are several reasons most often given for the need to have an abortion. They range from truly ridiculous to truly serious. I wish I could tell you that every time an abortion is sought there is a very serious and compelling situation. This is what those who espouse abortion will tell you. Unfortunately, it isn't true. Some of the more popular reasons given for the abortion decision are lack of financial stability, inconvenient timing, lack of medical insurance, education, parental anger, disappointment or embarrassment, drugs, fear of a handicapped child, and rape. Very few abortions are obtained for reasons of serious health problems, rape, or incest.

Loo was 26 years old, married, lived in Beverly Hills, and was an art student. She told me how terribly inconvenient this child would be. Loo didn't even think she would tell her husband--she would just have the abortion and get rid of the problem. Besides, he would probably want the child! She said her husband was older and he had promised to send her to Europe the following September to continue her education. If she did have the baby she told me she would have a nanny and would be able to continue her education in this country, but Europe would probably be out. She talked a long time. I'm fairly sure she had an abortion. I wonder how Europe was.

When a woman tells me, as Loo did, "I won't be able to finish my education and I won't be able to travel. I was going to go to Europe next year!," (or a similar story) I am reminded of the Statue of Justice, herself. On one side of the famous scale is the pregnant woman's lifestyle, on the other side is her baby. Which scale holds the heavier weight of justice? Which side is more important? The answer that saddens and frightens me is that many, many people would give the weight to a woman's lifestyle!

The circumstances of Loo's education and travel plans being delayed would have been simply that, a delay. All that needed to be changed was her timetable.

The "inconvenient-timing" excuses given for an abortion are most disturbing. One young woman said she was getting married in three months, and it just would be too difficult. She could see herself getting pregnant the following August, but not

# Liberated Women

right at that moment. Another said that she needed to "live a little" first, that she was too young to be a mother. A mental picture of these women appears in my imagination: They are standing next to a long conveyor belt, and they are inspecting tomatoes. They pick one up now and again and they inspect and reject certain ones. Some finally choose, but a lot of the ladies run out of choices.

"But, madam, your unborn baby is not a vegetable! He or she is a living, breathing human being. That which you are carrying inside of you is a boy or a girl. Your child has a personality, a beating heart, and a functioning brain. He has arms and legs. He has value." How can a woman say that she will be willing to have a child in a few months or a year, when her child is here, right now, inside of her, near her heart. It's a myth that when the timing is right, so will everything else be right.

The other extreme of pregnant women, not pregnant by choice, are among the heroines I have known--as in the case of Angie, the 13-year old, who was raped by a stranger, or Hannah, who became pregnant after being raped by a man she knew.

Hannah was blind, lived alone, but was helped by friends and her church community during her pregnancy. I was struck by the fact that neither the subject of abortion or self-pity ever came up in our conversations. This is what had had happened to her; she was in shock and sad, but she was dealing with it. I loved her, even though all of our conversations were by phone. One of our counselors did visit her and brought her some maternity and baby clothes. I subsequently met someone who knew her, a member of Hannah's church. She told me that Hannah had done well with the pregnancy and that her church had been there for her, with as much help as they could give. She gave the baby to loving, adoptive parents that she had chosen.

As I mentioned earlier, very few relationships survive an abortion. A Melissa will often tell me she will lose a Kevin or a John if she doesn't have the abortion. I try to tell her that once she has the abortion, she will change her mind about Kevin or John, anyway. He has supported or actively promoted the death of her child. And, even though she told herself that a seven-week unborn child was only a blob, a fetus, and that she was only having a "procedure," the reality of that child and the fact that it was *her* child hits her soon after the abortion with grief and guilt.

To say that women *don't* have abortions lightly, as a convenience, is a lie! The following are some of the more popular rationalizations we hear for abortion: "My mother and father will kill me;" "My boyfriend will leave me;" "I won't be able to finish my education;" "The timing is bad, I just got this job;" "I couldn't carry the baby for nine months and then give it up for adoption;" "If I knew who the father was, I might keep it (if it was the right man)."

These situations, although not entirely frivolous, still can't qualify as being as important as the life of another human being. These are all circumstances that will change or might not even materialize. For example, parents do not usually kill their daughters when they get pregnant. They might be angry, disappointed and hurt. There might be a temporary estrangement, but there probably would not be violence, unless there had already been a history of physical abuse in the family. More than likely, after the initial shock wears off, parents will still love and stand by their daughters.

In an overwhelming number of cases the young women we see have been in a dysfunctional home with a single-parent, or alcoholic-parent. The need for them to find a "Daddy" to love them has led them to early sexual experiences. Thirty years ago, the societal and familial disdain for unwed motherhood would have stopped them from engaging in pre-marital sexual intercourse, but the combination of their unstable families and the social peer pressures to have early sexual partners makes it almost impossible to go against the tide!

The violence, neglect, or lack of love that they have experienced in their families has subconsciously led them to seek love and acceptance in destructive ways--with drugs, alcohol or sex with near-strangers. Why would anyone think that another destructive act, the act of abortion, would cure these problems? Just imagine that, with a little help, the young mother can give life to her child. And, both during the pregnancy and afterward, she can be helped to create a better life for herself.

The best scenario for young teen mothers would be for

them to give their children to loving, adoptive parents--and then to get on with their lives. But getting on with their lives in a different way: by defining some positive goals with help from adults, (in their families or with professional counseling, if necessary). They would do this by facing the fact that there are consequences to sexual involvement. The pain of giving up their children is a very real one, but it will prove to be a positive influence in their lives, not a destructive one.

However, the pain of the loss of the child in abortion leads to feelings of guilt, grief, and a return to the destructive elements in their lives or the beginning of a negative way of living that can include alcoholism, drugs, eating disorders, depression, promiscuousness--a general disorder in lives that they can't get into focus.

Ninety-five percent of the women I have talked to who had an abortion did not continue the relationship with the boyfriend. If she has the abortion and her boyfriend sticks with her, she will sooner or later break off with him, anyway. The relationship does not stand up to the tumultuous change in this woman's life. She has been emotionally abandoned by the father of her child, sometimes by her parent or parents, and then she abandons her baby. These are heavy circumstances to deal with. She usually comes out of it with deep, and sometimes repressed, resentment and anger. She's angry with her boyfriend, her parents, and others involved in her abortion experience.

I do understand why young girls and women think, initially, that an abortion will be the only answer to their problem (even though it isn't the positive, moral, or life-giving solution). I understand how they come to the conclusion that it is the *only* way to go. The pressures to have an abortion are almost overwhelming. They find out too late that the traumatic experience of the abortion and its aftermath is uniquely their experience. They are in this all alone. Their families, boyfriends, husbands, friends, doctor and the media cannot help them afterwards. It was their children, their bodies and their decisions.

Regarding the trauma of the abortion experience, Colmin McCarthy quotes Fogel in his Commentary in the *St. Paul Sunday Pioneer Press* in 1971:

*"Fogel does not claim that mental illness automatically follows abortion. Says he: 'Often the trauma may sink into the unconscious and never surface in the woman's lifetime. But it is not as harmless and casual an event as many in the pro-abortion crowd insist. A psychological price is paid. I can't say exactly what. It may be alienation, it may be a pushing away from human warmth, perhaps a hardening of the maternal instinct. Something happens on the deeper levels of a woman's consciousness when she destroys a pregnancy. I know that as a psychiatrist."* [6]

The realities of the abortion experience include the facts that a woman experiences psychological damage and deep emotional pain, and her unborn child is not given a chance to experience anything! His life was taken from him before he had a chance.

In most cases, the women I have talked to who are considering an abortion or already have had one or more, do not value or respect themselves. They tell themselves that they are victims of circumstances, rather than free individuals who can overcome and control what seem to be insurmountable problems. This devaluation of themselves usually started long before they got pregnant, "by mistake." Very often they did not get pregnant completely without intent, but once their subconscious wish became a fact, they were too insecure to carry through with the pregnancy. The pressure from their boyfriend or their families was too much. If a young woman has grown up with a sense of self-respect, she makes good decisions and doesn't get pregnant, or if she does get pregnant, she makes good, life-giving positive decisions then, too.

When I ask young women if they would consider adoption for their unborn children, they almost all invariably say, "I couldn't carry a baby for nine months and then give it up." Embodied in this thinking is the rationalization that they are not mothers already, the lie that they have not bonded with that child at this point. The truth of the matter is that they carry within them their child, and whether they carry her for nine months or they destroy her at six weeks, they are mothers already, and there are permanent consequences from their abortion decision.

I understand the difficulty of giving up a child to another family, another mother. And I have come to understand how a

# Liberated Women

woman thinks she won't be affected by the unseen child, the unremembered abortion. It took me a long time to realize, however, that what they were really saying was: "If I don't see the baby, or know what it feels like to hold him, then I won't have any bad memories; I won't feel loss, grief or regret. If I have the abortion now, there won't be a problem!" Little do they know how wrong they are.

I know from my experience with pregnant women that the giving part in an adoption is a healthy choice that allows a woman to go on with her life, to begin a new beginning. No one will say that it won't be difficult, but it will be the better of the choices, the most positive, life-affirming answer.

Liberated women or liberated men? The only ones who have been liberated in all of these cases are the men, "saved" from responsibility and inconvenience. Women have not been freed by abortion; they have been entrapped and damaged by a lie.

Women will only be truly free when they rely on themselves to be independent decision-makers, compassionate and loving, but not taken in by the next man who comes along or the good girlfriend who tells them an abortion is the only way out. Women will be truly liberated when they discover their own self-worth is what they make it, (with or without a man) and that a loving family consists of a man and woman who love each other enough to marry and then to have children within that marriage.

---

[1] Susan Faludi, *Backlash: The War Against American Women*, Crown Publishers, Inc., NY, 1991, p. 403.

[2] Ibid.

[3] Carole A. Wilk, *Career Women and Childbearing*, Van Nostrand Reinhold NY, 1986, p. 22.

[4] Helen Gurley Brown, *Sex and the Single Girl*, Geis, NY, 1962.

[5] Colmin McCarthy, "A Psychological View of Abortion." *St. Paul Sunday Pioneer Press*, and From the *Washington Post*, March 7, 1971, as quoted in *Abortion & Social Justice*, Hilgers & Horan, Sun Life, Thaxton, Va., 1972, p. 76.

[6] Ibid.

# *Looking for Daddy: Where in the World is Mom?*

"The percent of children living in single-parent homes has more than tripled in the last three decades. Today, 17 million children live in single-parent homes." Approximately 90 percent of single-parent homes are homes without a father." _____William J. Bennett[1]

The intrusion of the sexual revolution and feminist ideology into the American family has contributed greatly to separation, divorce, and *living-together* arrangements, where the father is usually not a daily part of his children's lives. Single motherhood, where Dad left before his child was born, is so common that the traditional, two-parent family is difficult to find. The emotional damage and the beginnings of an unstable or dysfunctional lifestyle, including very early sexual activity for young girls without a father, is a familiar result.

When I see a young woman who tells me that she began to be sexually active when she was very young, almost always there can be found in her family's background either alcoholism, drug abuse, molestation, or incest. When girls begin having sex as young as 14 or 15, sometimes even earlier, they seem to be subconsciously seeking the father they never had. Most often, these sex-based episodes of romantic love or one-night stands became a way of life for them. They never find a relationship based on real love and mutual respect. They are missing a caring, interested father, and they seek love, approval, and acceptance wherever they can find it.

Very often, they have never known their fathers. Others have experienced physical or sexual abuse by their fathers or their mother's boyfriends. Alcoholic fathers are lost to their daughters as truly as the dads who aren't physically there. Others, who live with their divorced mothers, do know where their fathers are, but have only occasional interaction with Dad, and that often is not stable or loving. This search for Daddy is not consciously perceived by the girls themselves, but drives them toward early sex, unstable, short-term relationships or drug and alcohol abuse.

There seems to be a commonality among young women looking for Daddy in that they are almost always ready to forgive their fathers, either for his absence, his abuse or his disinterest. They often find another man or several men like him.

# Looking for Daddy

I will never forget the bizarre story (and I have no reason not to believe her) of a young woman who had left Texas to get away from her father. He had sexually and physically abused her for several years. She told me that he had murdered her sister, and gotten away with it. She knew that she had to stay as far away as possible from him in order to preserve her life and her sanity. But, <u>she defended him several times during our counseling session, saying that it wasn't really his fault.</u> I tried not to gasp!

She was looking for Daddy every time she had a new affair with an older man. She had had many and various by the time she was 21 years old. The thing that I hoped for her, was that she wouldn't find anyone even remotely like her father.

There are so many stories of young men and women living with their mothers alone. Where has Daddy gone? There are, of course, many different reasons for his absence, but it is usually divorce, alcoholism, abandonment, or a mother who has always been a single mom (and possibly has had several dads for her children).

A conservative estimate of the number of young women that I see in the Pregnancy Counseling Clinic who live in a two-parent, stable family is probably one percent. When a young woman tells me her particular story, I always ask about her current living arrangements. She is most likely to be living with her mother, or with Mom and Mom's boyfriend, or, if she is in her late teens or early twenties, living with her own boyfriend. Her father is most often not actively involved in her life or not around at all.

There is a pronounced difference between a family life that includes Dad and one that does not. The decisions and results when an unmarried girl in a two-parent, stable family gets pregnant and has her baby are also markedly different from the young woman who has never really known her father. Two young 16-year olds' stories are good examples of the contrast in homes where fathers were present or absent.

Michaelann came to us when she was 16 and pregnant by her 17-year old boyfriend, David. She was living with her mother and older brother. Her mother, separated from her husband, had just obtained a restraining order to keep Michaelann's father away from herself and the family. He had been physically abusing his wife and son for a long time.

Michaelann was also being abused, but not by her father. Her brother, Robert, had been beating her for two or three years. When she came to see us for a pregnancy test, she had a black eye from a recent beating. He said he was mad at her because she was still seeing her boyfriend. Robert didn't know at the time that she was pregnant by that boyfriend. Michaelann was afraid that when he found out, he would hurt her again, or David. In order to avoid the threat of additional beatings and to continue her education, Michaelann went to live in a maternity home until the baby was born.

Shortly after she had the baby, I called her. I was surprised to find that she had decided to live with her father and her new daughter. She told me that she had always been Daddy's favorite and he had never hurt *her*, so she moved in with him. I was surprised, also, that she would want to live with the man who had hurt her mother so often. Subconsciously, Michaelann is looking for the father she hopes is there. I'm afraid I'm skeptical about this hope, and skeptical about her ever finding stability in a two-parent household, where she is the parent.

> *"In a national sample, teenage women who grew up in a two-parent household were less likely to be sexually experienced, and thus at less risk of pregnancy, than adolescents in a single-parent household."*[2]

Of course, some teens do get pregnant while living with both parents, where they are not abandoned by their boyfriends and family when the pregnancy becomes known, but it isn't the norm. One girl we helped did fit into that category.

Cheryl had a father and family who supported her when she needed them. They certainly weren't thrilled about her getting pregnant when she was eighteen, but they knew that she was a promising student who held several scholarships and was headed for college, hoping to be a teacher, like her Dad Her parents, at first, wondered if she had ruined her life. But they accepted and helped her in this difficult situation. They were there for her during the pregnancy, and after.

Shortly after Cheryl had her baby girl, I called to chat. She said she had not made any long-term plans with her daughter's father. She said, "He talks about getting a job and going back to school." But Cheryl wasn't sure she believed him. She also told me that she had not resumed a sexual relationship with him and doesn't intend to. She was very ambivalent about their future together, but she was very positive about her plan to continue her education in the Fall. She hadn't had to search for Daddy or Mom. They were always there for her. She was one of the lucky ones.

Barbara Dafoe Whitehead wrote an article that was published in *The Atlantic Monthly* in April of 1993. It was a sellout. The article, "Dan Quayle Was Right," discussed at length what our disconnected families are doing to our children.

> *"Half of all marriages now end in divorce. Following divorce, many people enter new relationships. Some begin living together. Nearly half of all cohabiting couples have children in the household."* [3]

When families are so inter-mixed in their relationships, (Mom's boyfriend lives in, Dad's girlfriend is taking us out for dinner, Dad's girlfriend's son is now living here with us) young girls and teen boys are terribly confused about where they fit into the scheme of things. Who shall I be loyal to? Where will I live next weekend? What did I do wrong? Why did Dad leave? How do I act toward Dad's girlfriend?

Also, in her article, Barbara Whitehead quotes Victor Fuchs, a Stanford economist:

> *"But parents in disrupted families have less time, attention, and money to devote to their children. The single most important source of disinvestment has been the widespread withdrawal of financial support and involvement by fathers. Maternal investment, too, has declined, as women try to raise families on their own and work outside the home. Moreover, both mothers and fathers commonly respond to family breakup by investing more heavily in themselves and their own personal and romantic lives."* [4]

Another study, *The Index of Leading Cultural Indicators*, regarding single-parent households concluded the following:

> *"Controlling for factors such as low income, children growing up in [single-parent] households are at a greater risk for experiencing a variety of behavioral and educational problems, including extremes of hyperactivity and withdrawal; lack of attentiveness in the classroom; difficulty in deferring gratification; impaired academic achievement; school misbehavior; absenteeism; dropping out; involvement in socially alienated peer groups, and the so-called 'teenage syndrome' of behaviors that tend to hang together--smoking, drinking, early and frequent sexual experience, and in the more extreme cases, drugs, suicide, vandalism, violence, and criminal acts."* [5]

And, from the *New York Times'* December 26, 1992, edition, comes an article entitled "The Controversial Truth:

Two-Parent Families Are Better:"

> "*According to Rutgers University professor of sociology David Poponoe, 'in three decades of work as a social scientist, I know of few other bodies of data in which the weight of evidence is so decisively on one side of the issue: on the whole, for children, two-parent families are preferable.'*"[6]

A mother trying to balance a job, an ex-husband, a boyfriend, expenses, and the needy psyche of her 14- or 15-year old daughter would have to be a physical and emotional miracle worker to support, discipline, guide, and demonstrate her love for this girl, all on her own. The stability usually found by living in the same house and neighborhood for long periods of childhood are not even present as stabilizing factors for our young people.

> "*One study shows that about 38 percent of divorced mothers and their children move during the first year after a divorce. Even several years later the rate of moves for single mothers is about a third higher than the rate for two-parent families.*"[7]

Also, in her article, Barbara Whitehead points out that movies and television promote the untraditional, disrupted family, while increasingly portraying the two-parent family as a source of contempt and scorn--thinly disguised comedy. I must admit that I've only watched portions of it twice (I couldn't stomach anymore), but *Married With Children* is a prime example of scorn for the traditional family in the appearance of social satire. It is so cartoonish and so demeaning to normal families that any statement it might intend to make (giving it the benefit of the doubt that there is any purpose or message at all or that it is satire) is lost in an overflow of adolescent silliness--potty humor. Both Mom and Dad are ignorant louts, and the children aren't any better.
Michael Medved wrote about Hollywood's love affair with itself and its promotion of alternate lifestyles and values in his book, *Hollywood vs America*.

> "*...With Bart Simpson regularly turning up on lists of the most admired Americans, we've come a long way from the model of the hugely popular Andy Hardy movies of the 1930s, with young Mickey Rooney learning life lessons from his father (Lewis Stone), a stern but kindly small-town judge. If they remade those films today, it would be Andy who taught the old man a thing or two--about tolerance, or*

*environmentalism, or the joy of spontaneous sexuality, or new styles in hair or clothes, or the horrors of sexism or homophobia...*[8]

*"In today's climate, a television series called 'Father Knows Best' would be absolutely unthinkable--it would be deemed too judgmental, authoritarian, patriarchal, and perhaps even sexist. A program entitled 'Father Knows Nothing' would stand a far better chance."*[9]

Even movies made about two-parent families in the last few years have portrayed the father as a nitwit, weak-kneed wacko. In the movie, *Back to the Future*, which was basically delightful, I was always a bit uncomfortable with the depiction of the nerdy father saved by his more intelligent son. And, of course, we have great role-models in Homer Simpson and Fred Flintstone!

Unfortunately, just as alcoholism and drug addiction is often repeated in a family, so, also, is the high rate of single-momism, school drop-out rate and paternal abandonment. Even when it would seem evident to children how not to live their lives, they seem to continue the never-ending circle of dysfunctional living and instability.

I talked to a teacher recently at a local high school. She had been trying to help a young 17-year old, Hispanic girl, Maria. Maria shared in an Impact (peer counseling) Group the fact that she had a scheduled 12-week abortion, but couldn't come up with the rest of the money that she had to have in hand in order to go ahead with the procedure. She asked the counselor to loan her the money she needed. The counselor talked at great length with her. She discovered that Maria was living with her mother, an alcoholic stepfather, and three younger children whom she was mainly responsible for. She said that Maria feared her parents' reaction to her pregnancy. Maria was not even sure who the father of her unborn child was. She said she wished she had waited until she was married before she had had a sexual relationship. Obviously, Maria would have fared better had she lived in a family without an alcoholic stepfather that she feared. She probably would not have looked for love in the arms of several teen boys. I don't know what finally happened, but Maria's abortion would not solve her problem; it would just be added to her list of miserable experiences.

Sometimes, a poor or non-existent relationship with a woman's father in her childhood will discourage her from ever wanting to be a mother herself. Psychologist Carole A. Wilk did a study of several women careerists, who were trying to decide if and when to have children. In her book, *Career Women and Childbearing*,[10] she developed an interesting chart about those who were sure, not so sure, and definitely positive about starting or not starting a family. The A group was ambivalent, the B group positively wanted children, and the C group positively did not want children. She found that all of the group C women felt unloved or abandoned by their fathers!

One of her subjects, a top executive, who also was sure that she wanted children, is an example of a confident woman with a good marriage and career:

*"Let's now consider some elements of Barbara's identification with father. Her father read to her, did puzzles with her, supported her verbal development, and rewarded her for her accomplishments with his added attention. Furthermore, by his example, that is, by the fact that he regularly came in and out of the home environment without loss of love or family role--he became an ego resource and a safe behavior model."*[11]

What a wonderful model for all dads is Barbara's father. I'm willing to bet that he is still as interested and supportive of what Barbara does and thinks. He loves, respects and enjoys her, just as he does his son. He encourages her as a career woman and as an individual in her adulthood, just as he did when she was a child.

Unfortunately, Barbara's situation and childhood experience is the exception, not the rule. Feminism and the so-called sexual revolution has so fragmented the traditional, two-parent family that most young girls (and boys) are denied this type of relationship and confidence-building with their fathers or their mothers. To undo what has been *socially correct* for the last thirty years will probably take another thirty years. All of society is affected by the unstable family. In order to change individuals and families, solid value-based education and moral role models must permeate our schools, churches, and entertainment.

When Moms are back in their homes for their children's early years, at least, and when the Dads are there also, we can begin again to see whole children, children who don't have to give up childhood in order to either take care of their broken families or seek love and approval elsewhere.

True feminism celebrates men and women equally, as their individual abilities and talents are acknowledged. It does not engage in a struggle for power. It seeks equality and early childhood encouragement of female talents and abilities, just as it promotes the same for sons.

A return to love and respect for each other and for our children, with a willingness to sacrifice some of our momentary pleasures, for long-term relationships and growth, can go a long way toward establishing families that encourage their children to wait for sex until marriage, as well as encouraging our sons *and daughters* to pursue their full potential in their education or careers.

In "Looking for Daddy," girls should find him in their homes in a loving, caring, and interested relationship. It should be based on mutual love and respect. Dad should not only be there physically, but should guide his daughter, and, yes, even talk to her about sex, exhorting her to wait for marriage before having a sexual relationship. Is this really so difficult to do? Why not encourage her to be the best she can be in school, in her social and sports activities? Why not help her develop self-confidence, independence and self-respect? Is this really so terribly difficult?

Girls and women who have found Daddy at home have found themselves, and don't need to look on the streets or in the arms of an older man or a 15-year old boy. They don't need to figure out how to act toward Dad's live-in girlfriend or Mom's boyfriend.

But, where in the world is Mom? Even when she's there? Frederica Mathewes-Green, Vice-President for Communications with *Feminists for Life* presents the paradox of perceived sexual freedom that has developed alongside the advances women have made in their professional lives:

*"Re-emerging feminism was concerned chiefly with opening doors for women to professional and public life, and later embraced advocacy of sexual freedom as well. Participation in public life is significantly complicated by responsibility for children, while uncommitted sexual activity is the most effective way of producing unwanted pregnancies."*[12]

Many women now forego childbearing, even if they are married, to pursue their careers. Many, however, have it in mind to gain success and recognition in their chosen fields, and then to become moms at some future date, later on.

In another part of her study of married couples, who were waiting to have children, Carole A. Wilk, described in detail many couples' lives and the factors that surrounded their decisions whether or not to have children and when to have them.

> *"As was obvious from their surroundings, Barbara and Jim had grown accustomed to a living standard based on two good incomes. They are able to afford the condominium, to dine out frequently, to take regular vacations, and even to get away for weekends when their work permits.*
>
> *"Of course, said Jim, if we were to start a family, we'd probably have to do so by the time Barbara is about 30. Then everything would change. (Their target of age 30 reflects couples who postpone the birth of the first child until the wife is about 30 years old).*
>
> *Barbara has some friends who tell her that after the baby was born, they couldn't bear to leave the baby every day. If she does not go back to work, for example, for six months or a year, what would happen to her career.*
>
> *Barbara is quite aware of the reality that her employer will probably not wait an open-ended period of time until she feels her primary early mothering tasks are completed. There is no such thing as one extra-wide step on the career ladder, labeled FOR NEW MOTHERS. In fact, she knows that once she drops out for a substantial length of time, she will have a very tough time ever rising to the top--no matter how competent she is, or how enlightened the organization is."* [13]

Some women don't want to defer childbearing, but want to have it all, right now. They go ahead and have that "wanted" child, but return to their job or career soon after. What are the effects of leaving a child in day care after only 6 weeks or maybe even 6 months? Carole Wilk described in her book some research on the effects of mothers leaving their children in early childhood. In the late 1960's Mary Ainsworth, a psychologist, devised a laboratory experiment called the <u>Strange Situation</u>. By means of a two-way mirror, observation is made of a child alone with his mother and brightly colored toys. The psychologist comes in, briefly chats with the mother, and then his mother leaves. The mother comes back in three minutes. The reactions of the child are observed and noted. The patterns of reunion were categorized.

If the child readily moves toward his mother and wants to be held (objecting if his mother puts him down too soon), he displays a <u>secure attachment</u> pattern to his mother. He has found her overall consistently there, attentive and trustworthy in the past, and the short separation has not betrayed that trust.

The child of an inconsistent mother, one who is there for him sometimes and sometimes not, may react either passively or aggressively. This child is termed <u>anxious-resistant</u> in his attachment pattern. He might sob uncontrollably, or may react passively.

The child who is classed as <u>anxious-avoidant</u> has been consistently rejected by his mother. Either she has been unsure of her role as mother or too tired from her ten hours of work outside the home to give much physical solace or attention to her infant. This child will react by demonstrating a disinterested, independent demeanor. He builds up a wall that sometimes isn't even discovered until he is an adult. It's his way of protecting himself from a mother and others who don't seem to be interested in attachment with him.

The feminists of the 60's and today will say that the drudgery of staying home for women is not worth the results of the independent, confident, but relationally well-connected children that come out of that mother/housewife household. But, I say that if a woman looks beyond the drudgery and uses her innate qualities of imagination, intuition, and managing skills, she can put up with the *boring necessities* and be a loving, secure home-based human being for her children. Indeed, she can, with a little management that includes doing nurturing things for herself, make a home filled with joy for all. Her positive outlook is certainly made easier by a supportive, involved husband, but can be done without, if she has the self-confidence, desire and tenacity to do it.

If she can look at her life with a more expansive vision, she will be able to see that in just a few short years, maybe only three or four, her child will be willing and ready to leave her for several hours of the day. She can look forward to and plan for that time, or she can work in her home. There are many kinds of small businesses she could pursue there. In this age of telephones, computers, fax machines, etc. she does not have to be isolated or left out of business.

Again, in the article, "Dan Quayle Was Right," Mrs. Whitehead describes, unfortunately, what has happened to families as we go into the 90's:

> *"Motherhood no longer defines adult womanhood, as everyone knows; equally important is the fact that fatherhood has declined as a norm for men. In 1976 less than half as many fathers as in 1957 said that providing for children was a life goal. The proportion of working men who found marriage and children burdensome and restrictive more than doubled in the same period. Fewer than half of all adult Americans today regard the idea of sacrifice for others as a positive moral virtue."*[14]

There was a day, during the difficult, early childhood years when I almost "lost it" (my mind, that is). My eldest daughter was 5, my son was 2 years and 10 months and not potty trained, and my infant daughter, Sara, was just under 3 months. I had just changed two sets of dirty diapers, after cleaning up a lunch mess and before that picking up my kindergarten daughter from school. I ended up sitting in the bathroom on the floor, crying out and sobbing, "I can't take any more of this. This is just too much to ask of any one person. I am tired! Somebody help me!" I told my husband about the scene I had made, alone with my three children. Dear man that he is, he said and did what he could. He told me the next day that he had decided that he would, from then on, do all of the marketing. I was delighted. Little did he know that to this day that would be his job. Little did he know how well I would adapt to not shopping.

Luckily, I got through the next two months, somehow--when my son finally showed definite signs of not needing a diaper any longer, and I became a little physically stronger. I had bottomed out and my hysterical crying had been a good release. Life wasn't a piece of cake at that time. I could never tell anyone that that was easy. But, and this is a big *but*, I got through it and so did my children. I, of course, had no thought of going back to work, but I could have used some rest. If my Mom had been closer I might have asked her to give me a break once a week by taking one or more of the children, or if we had had the extra money I might have found a baby-sitter for a few hours one day a week. As I think back on it, I would have lived that time period a little differently. I'm a great believer in confronting a problem and trying to solve it, if possible. I know, however, that my looking for a job and trying to get away from my children ten hours a day was never even a brief, passing thought in my mind! Nor would it have been any kind of an answer for a difficult period. Anyone who thinks that Mom not being in the home for ten to twelve hours every day solves anything is looking for long-term problems with children that may not be fixable.

One of the common contributing factors in all of this family disruption and instability is the feminist emphasis on self-centered behavior for women.

*"Once the social metric shifts from child well-being to adult well-being, it is hard to see divorce and nonmarital birth in anything but a positive light."*[15]

# Looking for Daddy

A fulfilling, interesting career or job for Mom needn't be measured by how many dollars she makes. A successful career doesn't need to be full-time big-bucks. It should be enriching and satisfying, but should take into consideration all of the factors that contribute to a healthy, happy child and marriage. A great, part-time job may take awhile to find, but it's worth the search.

I would like to say that some women <u>can</u> do it all, simultaneously. Certainly they are the more super-human types, but I don't think most of us can. A deferred career <u>or</u> deferred parenthood is very possible, however. If a woman wants to establish herself first in her chosen field, so be it. And then, as many women in Wilk's study concluded, it will be time, around age 32 or so, to begin a family.

Women have an amazing capacity for creativity, endurance, sociability, and longevity. We should use these abilities for both worlds: home and parenting; or career and advancement in a chosen field. Each needs to be done separately, however, if either is to be done well. Mothers who choose motherhood only, need to be respected and admired for their contribution to their families, their children, and society, in general. And women who choose careers, but decide not to have children, should be admired as well. They make their contributions in other ways. Respect and admiration for their job well done simply comes from other sources than their families. And for all of the single women who are that way by choice or circumstance, their careers and the ways in which they live their lives should be honored, acknowledged, and respected, as well. I salute all who have had the insight to know which life is for them. And, to all women who haven't quite decided, or who have tried to do too much, or feel that they are unfulfilled, I say think about it very carefully before you make any decisions. Career and children go together well, but only in chronological order, not simultaneously.

Where is Daddy? Hopefully, he is at home for his wife and children. And, hopefully, he sees himself as more than the person who goes out every day to bring home the paycheck. And, where in the world is Mom? Hopefully, she is at home when she's needed and fulfilled there, and out working when it's time. Where are the children? Hopefully, they are in a home of stability and nurturing, where both Mom and Dad contribute to their spiritual, moral, and academic development-- a home with some sacrifice, some discord, some problems, but one where there is love and joy. That's where the true feminist men and women will come from, and that's where the stable, productive families of the future will come from.

---

[1] William J. Bennett, *The Index of Leading Cultural Indicators*, published jointly by Empower America, The Heritage Foundation, and Free Congress Foundation, Vol. I, March 1993, p. 15, and from U. S. Bureau of the Census, Current Population Reports, , p-20, No. 450, "Marital Status and Living Arrangements, 1991."
[2] C. D. Hayes, ed., *Risking the Future: Adolescent Sexuality, Pregnancy, and Childbearing*, Vol. I, National Academy Press: Wahington, D. C. 1987.
[3] Barbara Dafoe Whitehead, "Dan Quayle Was Right," article in the *Atlantic Monthly*, April 1993, p. 50.
[4] Ibid., p. 58.
[5] William J. Bennett, *The Index of Leading Cultural Indicators*, published jointly by Empower America, The Heritage Foundation, and Free Congress Foundation, Vol. I, March 1993, p. 15. And from Urie Bronfenbrenner, "Discovering What Families Can do," in *Rebuilding the Nest : A New Commitment to the American Family* , David Blankenhorn, Steven Bayme, and Jean Bethke Elshtain, eds. (Milwaukee: Family Service Agenda, 1990).
[6] Ibid.
[7] Barbara Dafoe Whitehead, "Dan Quayle Was Right," article in the *Atlantic Monthly*, April 1993, p. 58.
[8] Michael Medved, *Hollywood vs. America*, Harper Collins Publishers, NY, NY, 1992, p. 147.
[9] Ibid., p. 148.
[10] Carol A. Wilk, *Career Women and Childbearing*, Van Nostrand Reinhold/ NY 1986.
[11] Ibid., p. 9.
[12] , Frederica Mathewes-Green, "Abortion and Women's Rights," *ALL About Issues Magazine*, American Life Lobby, March-April 1992, p. 13.
[13] Carol A. Wilk *Career Women and Childbearing*, Van Nostrand Reinhold/ NY 1986 pp. 4 & 5.
[14] Barbara Dafoe Whitehead "Dan Quayle Was Right," by article in the *Atlantic Monthly*, April 1993.
[15] Ibid.

# *Sex Before Sixteen*

"Today there is more brutal violence and explicit sex on television than ever before."[1]

_____Index of Leading Cultural Indicators

While interviewing Frederica Mathewes-Greene, I asked her if she could think of a role model for young women. She came up with Brooke Shields, who has publicly stated that she will remain a virgin until she is married, and I came up with A. C. Greene of the Los Angeles Lakers, who, obviously is a good model for young men, but I couldn't see my daughters having as a role model a male, professional basketball player. A. C. said in an interview appearing in *Focus on the Family* Magazine.

*"Sex itself isn't bad. It's just a matter of when to experience it. God created it for enjoyment, but He also reserved it for marriage. So I'm waiting."*[2]

After my conversation with Frederica, I tried to think of other famous female individuals who might publicly proclaim such "radical" ideas as waiting for a sexual relationship until they are married. I could come up with plenty of Barbara Streisands or Sybill Shepherds. Or, how about Madonna? Now there's a terrific role model for our daughters. But, I wasn't able to recall any other female entertainment or sports figure who had publicly declared herself in favor of waiting for sex until marriage. I certainly hope there are some shy types out there who think that way, but just aren't ready to come forward. At any rate, A.C. Greene is certainly on my list of heroes. Magic Johnson, a much-loved basketball hero, when he found out he had AIDS, (acquired immune deficiency syndrome) missed a golden opportunity for teaching young people to wait for marriage. Instead, he preferred to be fashionable, and politically-correct by promoting condoms as a safe-sex resource. It would have been better for all of us if he had had the courage to promote abstinence before, and fidelity during, marriage.

What our young people are treated to after school, for homework, is "love in the afternoon," via the current brand of soap operas (jump in bed first, question later) or titillating talk shows. I heard just yesterday on a radio commercial that Geraldo is going to have some gentleman on his show who will submit to a sex-change operation right before our very eyes! In the name of liberation and sexual sophistication, some of the most bizarre behavior is highlighted and presented as interesting fare for a lazy afternoon. I happened to turn on the Montel Williams Show[3] one afternoon and was treated to a display of eight women who called themselves the Sex Sluts. The owner of the Ecstasy Lounge, a lesbian nightclub and self-entertainment establishment, located somewhere near San Francisco, was explaining how expensive it was for her to keep her customers happy. "Well, you know we have to have condoms, lube, futons..." I learned that they are very careful about "safe sex" in their club.

Some of the women, who were most remarkably dressed, spoke about their involvement. One, a petite Filipina woman, said that she was a stripper and that she preferred doing it for women, rather than for men. She said that her strict, Catholic, cultural background had been very restrictive, and now she feels really free when she does her act. All I could think of was her mother. Does she know? How does she feel? All I could hope for was that her mother still lived in the Phillipines, never sees Montel Williams, and that her daughter lies to her about what she does for a living. This was an obviously sick, but attractive, young woman who was being used by other women and Montel Williams and his producers. My aversion to such trash invading my home turned quickly to pity for these women, who obviously needed help. But, it didn't change the fact that this perversion was openly available to my children.

I will never forget my feelings of shock when I learned from my 13-year-old daughter that KROQ radio in Los Angeles, regularly features late-night programming that discusses homosexual activities. When she asked me about anal beads, and I said, "What?", she repeated it and told me that they were used for sexual stimulation! I'm afraid I took the coward's way out. I told her about my feelings of revulsion and outrage, but said I didn't think I could stomach anymore information. This program had been on about 10:00 PM the night before.

Though I prefer other types of music, I decided to listen to KROQ the following Saturday afternoon. Surely, this would not be so sensational--in the daytime? Wrong! Not! What I heard was a disk jockey and a young girl and her mother discussing what happens in intercourse. It was a cute little contest, you see. She was supposed to describe a certain action and effect, and then get her mother to give the correct answer over the air. The young girl asked her Mom, "What is it when a boy puts his penis in a girl's vagina and it gets wet?" Her eminently intelligent mother answered, "Do you mean lubrication?" I turned the radio off, never finding out if they won $10, $1000 or just the Dumb Bunny Award for participating. I was simply too shocked and saddened. If this kind of garbage reaches hundreds of thousands of teens daily, just in the Los Angeles. area, why are we shocked with promiscuity, sexual experimentation, and unwed pregnancies before teens are 15?

The liberal answer about our being able to turn off offensive programming is such a joke. "Parents should know what their children are doing, what they are listening to and watching--at all times of the day and night." Is that what liberalism means, that we lock up our radios and televisions, that we send a bodyguard or *duenna* to school with our kids? There is simply no way to avoid this senseless trash unless we put one of those prison ankle-bracelet sensors on our children. This is freedom? I call this kind of televised perversion for entertainment an invasion of my privacy.

What is never mentioned on the sexy soaps are some of the devastating results of sexual promiscuity. Very often, a woman will become pregnant in the storyline, but have you ever seen, after the thrilling *slo-mo* sex scene, a man or woman saying "Oh, oh, I'd better go to the doctor for an STD (sexually transmitted disease) test. I'm not feeling too well." When has Tom Hanks, or Tom Cruise, or Tom anybody ever come up with a very realistic disease from his night or nights with his female co-star?

Years ago, there were only two venereal diseases to worry about: gonorrhea and syphilis. Now there are six:

Chlamydia is the most widespread in the U. S. It is a bacterial infection that can be cured with antibiotics. However, its symptoms aren't apparent until serious complications arise. It can lead to pelvic inflammatory disease (PID), which can cause chronic pain, tubal pregnancies, and infertility or sterility.

Herpes has increased greatly in recent years. It is, of course, a virus and is not curable. The symptoms can be treated, but, while active, they are very unpleasant, including: sores on the sex organs; fever; enlarged lymph glands; and flu-like symptoms. There are continuing outbreaks of this disease, and if a child contracts it in delivery he may become seriously ill or die.

Human papilomavirus (HPV) is commonly known as genital warts. It, like herpes, is a virus (incurable) spread by direct sexual contact with the warts. They appear singly or in clusters on or around the genitals or anus about one to three weeks after infection. It is particularly dangerous to women because it has been found in almost all cancers of their reproductive organs.

Gonorrhea is a bacterial infection that can be treated with antibiotics. Women may develop a vaginal discharge. Gonorrhea can lead to PID, infertility and crippling arthritis.

Syphilis affects 16 percent of our population. It is a bacterial infection and can be treated if it is diagnosed early. It produces an infectious sore called a chancre. In women it can be internal. After one to five weeks the sores will disappear, be followed by a rash and a weak, tired feeling. However, if left untreated, it can be a deadly disease. Other results, if untreated, include blindness, heart disease, nervous disorders, insanity, tumors and death. An unborn child can contract this disease during pregnancy.

Acquired Immune Deficiency Syndrome (AIDS) is a killer with no cure, at present. It is estimated that one and a half million people are infected with HIV, the virus that causes AIDS. It is spread through sexual contact and blood to blood contact. There are no symptoms at first and it may take five to ten years to appear after the initial infection. Because the immune system is attacked, people infected with this disease contract many different health problems, including respiratory infections, heart and nervous disorders. Treatments available now only postpone death.

I had two 14 year-old girls in my office the other day. They both wanted pregnancy tests. I asked them if they weren't worried about getting a sexual disease. They both giggled and answered, "No." I asked if they knew if their older boyfriends had been with other girls sexually. They both said yes, but they weren't worried.

The Alan Guttmacher Institute, known as the educational arm of Planned Parenthood, decided to conduct research on teens to find out why they had such poor contraceptive practices. In 1983, the researchers began ten discussion groups with teens in Chicago, Indianapolis, Janesville, Wisconsin, New York City and Seattle. The results, I fear, were not what the Institute would like to have heard, but the truth is difficult to hide. So, they ignored the obvious. Their analyses and suggestions for teens were outrageous, especially in light of their findings.

Their pre-established agenda included more condoms and more pills, not chastity and self-control. Here are some of the teens' comments:

# Sex Before Sixteen

*"My girlfriend had just gotten pregnant, and she kept telling me she was sexually active and she didn't have a steady boyfriend, but she was sleeping around with different guys that she dates, and she wouldn't get on the birth control pill. She was on it one time, but quit it right away. And she ended up pregnant. And right away she just got an abortion. And now she's sitting at home regretting that she got an abortion."*[4].

*"I know a girl who has had a few abortions. She was in the 9th grade, and she's in 10th now. Two girls I know had more than two or three."*[5]

Some of Planned Parenthood's analyses of these situations included the fact that kids are given double messages in movies, television, magazines, etc. One message is that sex before marriage is bad. The other extols the "virtues" of being and acting sexy. To be cool is <u>not</u> to be a virgin.

I agree that kids are given the sexy message, but I don't see the abstinence or "no sex before marriage" message anywhere. Where did Planned Parenthood see it? Unfortunately, I don't think teens do get a double message--they don't hear about virginity, abstinence, and morals, and <u>especially not</u> from Planned Parenthood. Here is one of PP's comments on the study. One would think that the obvious modesty noted in teens might be natural and encouraged by this organization. Not so.

*"They are shy, ill at ease, and self-conscious when they find themselves about to have sex for the first time with a new partner, when dealing with parents reluctant to learn about their children's burgeoning sexual feelings, or when trying to buy a contraceptive product from the local druggist."*[6]

Their answer, instead, is this:

*"Teenagers who have had satisfactory experiences obtaining services should be used in broad information programs to publicize the fact that clinics and physicians don't squeal on their patients."*[7]

In other words, <u>We should use propaganda in the form of peer counseling to broaden the scope of the contraceptive message to teens, and let them know that they can get contraception and abortions without their parents' knowledge.</u> My answer would be to use peer counseling to promote the advantages and wisdom of morality, self-control, and self-awareness of what is valuable, life-giving behavior. I would also encourage them to go to their parents for advice, direction, and help. If theirs is a dysfunctional, unstable family, I would encourage them to go to a trusted relative or adult friend (someone over twenty-one). I would not encourage a trip to Planned Parenthood.

Planned Parenthood would most likely answer me with this quote from their literature:

> *"Programs to teach and encourage parents to communicate with their children about sexual matters are likely to have limited potential for improving the contraceptive practice of teenagers."*[8]

In other words, "Don't go to your parents, kids, they'll only ask you to behave yourself and treat you like children!" The really frightening directive that came from their analysis of this teen/contraceptive research is the following:

> *"A widespread campaign could be launched to inform doctors and teenagers that the pill is the safest as well as the most effective contraceptive method for most teenagers. The growing awareness of the risks of sexually transmitted diseases provides fertile ground for improving knowledge of the role the condom can play in preventing the spread of venereal infections."*[9] (Their use of the term, "fertile ground," is especially interesting.)

I disagree that the pill has been proven to be so safe. From all that I hear about symptoms and contraindications for its use from my clients (and how they got pregnant after they stopped taking it), I would be very careful in dispensing the pill if I were a physician. The wholesale giveaway that is promoted by Planned Parenthood, with no real medical follow-up for young women is frightening. Here is a statement made by Dr. Herbert Ratner in 1969.

> *"The American woman, both rich and poor, black and white, is being victimized by social engineers. Population control rather than the health of the individual has become the new directing force of the family planning movement..." "When preoccupation is with control rather than planning, people are viewed numerically as statistics, and concern for the welfare of the individual, the person, diminishes. An effective contraceptive rather than a safe one becomes prime consideration and the technological achievement replaces the humanistic goal. Despite the fact that we knew in advance that a powerful chemical disruptive of*

*normal physiological mechanisms was being introduced, The Pill has been the most poorly tested drug ever approved by the FDA...*"[10]

Birth control pills are handed out by Planned Parenthood to young teen girls, and children are given condoms like candy in school-based clinics. Clinics are supported by grants from pharmaceutical companies. I wonder why!

Since Dr. Ratner questioned the pill's safety in 1969, a new, long-term contraceptive has been developed, Norplant. It was discovered that nurses at San Fernando High, here in Southern California, were implanting this device into teen girls without their parents' knowledge. Never mind that the Norplant drug has not been sufficiently tested on teen girls, some of whom may not even have a regular menstrual cycle yet. The device, implanted in the girls' arms, interferes with their normal cycles. These young women are being experimented on without any long-term knowledge of side effects! And, nurses who insert the Norplant device are selling out their younger sisters by promoting this type of social engineering--most of the girls at this school are Hispanics.

Should it be offered at school clinics, as it was at San Fernando High? Should I offer it to my daughters? My girls are 23, 18, and 13. I pictured to myself what it would be like to have a discussion with them about Norplant and how it would go. I came up with two very different scenes: "Girls, I know that I've tried to raise you with values, but I also know that you're weak and irresponsible, unable to control your sexual urges. So, I have decided you should have Norplant. It's reversible, and for five years you can have sex with anyone and not worry about getting pregnant. You might have to worry, however, about sexually transmitted diseases. Despite what you may have heard in school or on television, condoms can't keep you safe from AIDS, chlamydia, or genital warts. But, don't worry. If you do get Norplant, then I, as your Mother, will not have to worry about being embarrassed if you get pregnant. I will appear modern and liberated. I will be your friend, and therefore I won't have to give you guidelines or rules for living. I won't have to be involved. I mean, really, you've had all kinds of sex education in school! I'm sure you know it all. In fact, I understand that KROQ has a wonderful radio show on at 10:00 PM where all kinds of sex is discussed in great detail. I know that you've learned a lot from the soaps on TV, too. Movies today are great at giving you an understanding of sexy people. You really don't need me, except to help you get fixed up with this implant thing that does something to your hormones."

Or—"I love you and value you as individuals who need to mature and develop into loving, whole young women who recognize your own self-worth, apart from, and including, your sexuality. When you get married you and your husband will be in a committed relationship that you share and nurture together, not just a relationship where you use one another in order to satisfy your sexual urges. I want you to know that you will be selling yourselves short if you get sexually involved before you are married. Others, like Planned Parenthood, feminists, school nurses, etc. want you to think that all you need is a condom or a pill, or now an implant, so that you can be liberated and there will be no evident consequences to your actions. But, let me tell you when you begin to be sexually active with one man or boy, or with several, at this time in your life, there are consequences. School will become less interesting and less important. Your grades and lifetime goals will be subconsciously out of the picture. You will be vulnerable to any STD that your partner has been exposed to. You will worry about his enduring love for you. And, you will see yourself as valuable only as long as you are in a sexual relationship."

I'd like to repeat my second scenario for all teens, boys and young men included. All need to hear about their intrinsic dignity and self-worth. They need to know that a sexual relationship, whether long or short-term at ages 14, 15, or even 18, does nothing for them in their individual development into adult man- or womanhood. It can only give them a false view of what sexuality really means in a committed, loving, married relationship. They need to know that there is more to life than being "with it," and that they can become leaders in their own youthful environment by saying "no" and making abstinence in high school the popular thing to do. I'd like to talk to the doctors and nurses who believe that promoting Norplant, condoms, and the pill is the moral, ethical, and necessary thing to do. What *are* you thinking about?

What about condoms for safe sex? A woman can get pregnant only about 36 days per year, but anyone can get AIDS 365 days per year. The AIDS virus is 410 times smaller than any sperm. A physician asked his audience at a medical seminar how many prescribed condoms as a preventive measure against the AIDS virus. All raised their hands. The doctor then posed the following question to his audience: "What if you meet someone at this convention, you're attracted by him or her and, even though there is a possibility that this person might have been exposed to this deadly disease, how many of you would use a condom and have an affair with this person?" There was not one hand raised in the audience. What's good enough (a condom) for the patient is not always good enough for the doctor!

With all of the hype and promotion about safe sex one would think that condoms are the be-all and end-all, so that we can do exactly what we feel like doing when the urge comes over us. Steven J. Sainsbury, a physician, wrote a column, printed in the *Los Angeles Times*, about condoms for kids:

*"...Condoms fail, and fail frequently. Due to improper storage, handling and usage by consumers, the condom breakage rate during vaginal intercourse is 14%. Other high-risk behaviors, particularly anal intercourse increase this rate significantly. For the person who averages sex three times a week, a 14% breakage rate equates to a condom failure every two weeks.*

*AIDS is a killer disease, and any measures taken to prevent its transmission must be used every time and can never break or leak. Neither criterion is ever likely to be met. Condoms may mean 'safer' sex, but is 'safer' acceptable for this deadly epidemic?"*[11]

We have seen at our clinic the results of twenty years of value-free education in our schools. When our young people seek guidance, they are given explicit sexual information on sexual intercourse and "outercourse."

The brainwashing that has proliferated with the likes of Planned Parenthood, school-based clinics, school boards, state education departments, the Sex Information and Education Council, and others, has stolen our children from us. Indeed, <u>they have stolen childhood from our children</u>. We parents need to take back our kids.

A long-term course in family values wouldn't hurt. Just what are these family values that I'd like to instill in my children? Is it just an overused term that is ridiculed by the liberal media? Or is it really something of substance, a basic way of living, something to be sought after and learned? Certainly, values aren't taught in our public schools. Kids in our public schools are taught sex and everything else in an amoral vacuum. The schools now own our children! God help us. God? Who's God?

Family values are ideals promoted by families where morals and religious beliefs are taught and lived out. When a boy or girl develops into adulthood with an underpinning of the ten commandments, he or she usually has a much better chance of avoiding the traumatic problems inherent in the use of drugs, alcohol, and sex. Generally, those who subscribe to family values will place a high priority on responsibility and consideration of others, both at school and at home. The family-values family will tell their children that sex before marriage is immoral and "not smart." Mom and Dad will try to instill in their children a healthy fear of hanging out with the wrong group, sexually transmitted diseases, and the dangers of drug and alcohol use.

William Kilpatrick did a thorough study of our education system, which he detailed in a recent book, *Why Johnny Can't Tell Right from Wrong.*[12]

*"The courts, for example, have decided that school prayer is not permissible even if students are not required to participate, because the very presence of prayer at school constitutes an implied endorsement of religion. In similar fashion, the presence of school-based clinics that pass out condoms would seem to lend legitimacy to sexual activity."*[13]

Say that again. The "legitimacy of sexual activity is promoted by clinics who pass out condoms?" Oh no, that isn't their purpose! Safety and sanity. Oh, yes, let's look at some of their kind of sanity:

*"Changing Bodies, Changing Lives, a text widely used in schools and recommended by the School Library Journal, is liberally sprinkled with quotes from teens describing their sexual experiences in minute detail. Fred, a gay student, relates, 'I was so excited the first time I had sex with a guy that I came just taking my pants off...' Donna, a seventeen-year-old, describes her experience: 'I was with this guy who said, 'Let me do something to you that I think you'll really like.' And that was when he went down on me and started licking me. I was really kind of embarrassed...But it felt really, really good, and I relaxed and just got into it.' At regular intervals the authors remind their young readers, 'There's no 'right' way or 'right' age to have life experiences, ' and 'only you can decide' what is right.'"*[14]

We have School Clinics where the nurses are willing to insert Norplant into the bodies of trusting teen girls who think they will be safe from pregnancy for five years with this device. At least these "ladies" can indulge in sexual relationships (how many different partners can they have in five years?) and be assured that they will not get pregnant. But, the physical and psychological effects will be monumental, and possibly irreversible! The pill can be obtained in the school clinics and abortions can be procured with the help of school counselors. All this can be done without parental consent or knowledge!

According to Planned Parenthood, who get into as many schools as they can:

> *"Sexual activity has increased among American adolescents since the early 1970's. The average age at first sexual intercourse is 17.2 for females and 16.5 for males. By age 20, three out of four females and five out of six males have had sexual intercourse."*[15]

What is Planned Parenthood's reactions to their own statistics? What is our educational system's answer to this news? "Here's a condom, learn how to have "safe" sex. Here is what female and male genitalia look like and how they operate during intercourse. Everyone must make his own decisions about sex. There is no right or wrong, whatever you are comfortable with."

And, this is how they propose to lower the pregnancy rate? How about some photos made into huge posters of vaginal warts or what chlamydia does to the human body? How about the medical risks of abortion and a picture of the instruments used to suck out unborn children from their mothers' wombs? How about pictures of aborted "products of conception." How about some truth, instead of fiction?

It seems that today's teens don't have a chance. If their parents aren't there to instill values or educate them about sex, because of overwork or broken families, they must rely on their teachers or counselors and their peers. They are taught in school that they need information to make them safe, but it must be neutral information because anything that sounds like a moral might be based on a religious ideology, and there must not even be a hint that religion even exists in this country.

If their parents are there and are trying to guide them, morally, then they are confused by receiving a different message from teachers, counselors, and friends. Today, forty-seven states formally require or recommend Sex Ed. All fifty support AIDS Education. Does this help or does this confuse our children? Again, James Kilpatrick, in his book, *Why Johnny Can't Tell Right from Wrong*, talks about the harm to teens that the values-free, safe-sex approach can produce.

> "But there is an even greater unreality lying at the bottom of the safe-sex approach, and that is the assumption that pregnancy and sexually transmitted diseases are the only problems. Another possibility--that one can do harm to one's personality as well as to one's health through casual sex--is largely ignored. The link between sex and character is a missing link in sex education.."[16]

Planned Parenthood does their thing with condoms and bananas, promotes the pill and secret abortions! How has it helped decrease sexual activity, STD's, and unwanted pregnancies? According to their own findings, sexual activity has increased among adolescents since the early 1970's, Twenty thousand girls drop out of school each year in California due to pregnancy and never finish high school.[17]

James Kilpatrick talks about abstinence education in the schools:

> "In 1981, with the passage of the Adolescent Family Life Act, federal funds became available for the development of abstinence-based curriculums. The bill was aimed at encouraging programs that would 'clearly and unequivocally' promote abstinence. It also called for greater family involvement in the development of programs, since 'prevention of adolescent sexual activity and adolescent pregnancy primarily depends upon developing strong family values and close family ties."[18]

What a unique idea--waiting for marriage, presenting sex as something to look forward to. Not so, for some. Mr. Kilpatrick continues,

> "But abstinence education was not warmly received by established sex educators. Instead, it was met with a great deal of opposition. Planned Parenthood; the Alan Guttmacher Institute; Education Training and Research; the Center for Population Options; and various other groups balked at the idea of abstinence. Michael Hall, a Planned Parenthood executive, spoke for many when he warned that 'teens will be totally turned off.' Meanwhile, just in case teens didn't react in the proper way, the AFLA was challenged almost yearly in Congress, and its programs were resisted on the state and local level. The American Civil Liberties Union even filed suit against the AFLA [Adolescent Family Life Act (1981) on the grounds that the promotion of abstinence constituted an establishment of religion."[19]

To not even encourage young people to be chaste (abstinent), but conclude ahead of time that they have no

# Sex Before Sixteen

self-control, no idea of respect for each other or the dignity of each human person is demeaning to all of them. It's laziness on the part of the parents and it's indoctrination on the part of educators who believe in sex education without a moral base. Those parents who do encourage condoms and sex education in their schools, are saying, *"We don't want to deal with your teenage sex problems--just don't give us any grief by getting pregnant."* The educators are saying, *"We must educate (indoctrinate) these students, so that they will accept our agenda. It's so easy to do it here in school. They can become free thinkers (free to think what we teach them)."* The parents who give up and let the schools do the sex educating are essentially abandoning their children at the same time that their hearts and minds are being pursued by liberal teachers and liberal organizations.

Planned Parenthood has been active here in California, and the rest of the country, for a long time. Obviously, what they are doing has not worked! In one of their fact sheets, they tell us (very carefully avoiding any kind of boasting) that the teen birth rate decreased with the legalization of abortion. They also state, but never draw any logical conclusions, that:

*"Adolescents who initiate sexual intercourse at younger ages are more likely to have multiple partners in their adolescent years, thus increasing their chances of acquiring a STD, including HIV."*[20]

The type of feminism that suggests that teen girls should use condoms, pills, or Norplant to be safe does not protect, teach, improve or liberate them. It's a lie, a very dangerous lie, every time a teacher says that there is no right or wrong, or every time a Planned Parenthood counselor says, "The doctor will see you now; after your abortion you won't have anything to worry about." Our kids are used and abused. Our teen girls are told they aren't valuable unless they are sexy and lose their virginity early. They are also given the message that you are safe if you practice birth control, rather than self-control. Setting up this kind of thinking, as early as the third or fourth grade, robs our children of their natural sexual and social development. This inordinate emphasis on sex is not promoting values, wholeness, or safety. It's truly frightening.

Our young people are impacted by feminism subliminally, by sexual libertarians overtly, and by the overall lie of liberation from sexual responsibility. And that influence has proven to be a colossal failure.

We, at the Clinic, are always amazed at the teens who still don't think they will be the ones to get pregnant and have no fear of sexually-transmitted diseases. Their innocence and fearlessness would be delightful if it weren't so tragic. To say that our young people can't control themselves is insulting, at the very least. And when schools, parents and Planned Parenthood encourage condoms, the pill, abortion, (everything but abstinence), it's difficult for our youth to find out the truth about chastity before marriage: that it is possible and desirable.

Condoms do not protect them from sexually transmitted diseases, including AIDS, nor are they foolproof as a pregnancy preventative. The pill has side effects that many women do not tolerate well. And, if they have abortions, young women live a lifetime of regret or they try to get pregnant soon after, in order to make up for the child lost in the abortion.

Sex is no longer taught to our children as something that is part of God's plan to continue the human race and create loving, nurturing families. They are taught that it's a game, a device to be used for entertainment. Our children are exposed to so much trash, so much deviant sex that how any of them survives and enters into a caring, responsible relationship that might eventually lead to a stable marriage is beyond me.

It has been popular since the sixties for young people to scorn a marriage license as simply a piece of paper. Hopefully, very soon our young adults will find out the real truth about liberated lifestyles and begin to seek the more traditional arrangement, i. e., sex with their own husbands and wives in a committed, loving relationship.

Our young people, especially our young women, need to learn about the dignity of a real relationship between a man and a woman. If the abstinence/chastity message truly gets through to them, they will experience teen years full of fun and learning, maturing gradually. They won't always be looking for the next thrill and bored if they don't get it. Or anxious about their current "relationship." Or worried about a late menstrual period or symptoms of a sexually transmitted disease. They need to know that waiting for a loving, committed marriage is worth the self-discipline now, so that they can give themselves to their spouses as a whole person, one not damaged by abortion, disease, or a promiscuous lifestyle.

I love my country and what it used to stand for. But our country will have no future without healthy, stable, and responsible children. They won't be healthy if they are taught to choose condoms instead of self-control. They won't be stable if they don't learn that two people committed to one another in marriage is an ideal to strive for, and they won't be responsible if their "little mistakes" (their unborn children) are aborted for convenience.

---

[1] *Index of Leading Cultural Indicators*, published by Empower America, The Heritage Foundation, Free Congress Foundation, Vol. 1, March, 1993, cited from U. S. Dept. of Justice, Bureau of Justice Statistics, "Lifetime Likelihood of Victimization" Technical Report, March 1987, p. 20.
[2] "Fatherhood? Not Yet," in *Focus on the Family Magazine*, Focus on the Family, Colorado Springs, June 1993.
[3] *Montel Williams Show*, KCOP-TV, Los Angeles, 3/17/93.
[4] *Family Planning Perspectives*, Alan Guttmacher Institute vol. 17, no. 2, March, April 1985, p. 85.
[5] Ibid.
[6] Ibid., p. 89.
[7] Ibid.
[8] Ibid.
[9] Ibid.
[10] Herbert Ratner, M.D., "The Medical Hazards of the Birth Control Pill," *Child and Family Reprint Booklet*, published by Child and Family Quarterly Magazine, Oak Park, Illinois, 1969.
[11] Steven J. Sainsbury, M.D., "Condoms for Kids? Get Real,", *Los Angeles Times,* July 13, 1993, Section B, p. 13.
[12] William K. Kilpatrick, *Why Johnny Can't Tell Right from Wrong*, Simon & Schuster, NY, 1992.
[13] Ibid, p. 59.
[14] Information Sheet, Public Affairs Department, Planned Parenthood Los Angeles.
[15] Ibid.
[16] James Kilpatrick, *Why Johnny Can't Tell Right From Wrong*, Simon & Schuster, NY, 1992 pp. 62 & 63.
[17] Information Sheet, Public Affairs Department, Planned Parenthood Los Angeles.

[18] James Kilpatrick, *Why Johnny Can't Tell Right From Wrong*, Simon & Schuster, NY, 1992, p. 73.
[19] Ibid.
[20] C. S. Weisman, et al., "AIDS Knowledge, Perceived Risk and Prevention Among Adolescent Clients of a Family Planning Clnic," *Family Planning Perspectives (FPP)*, Sep/Oct 1989.

# The Media, Feminism and Abortion

"To begin with Bernie, we're not tax-deductible, being political, so we can't spend a lot of money on PR. We have to create our own publicity, which means demonstrations, disruption, lawsuits, and a ruthless courting of the press and the TV. Most of the young women reporters for the big papers and TV are committed to our cause, especially here in the East where the media are, and we really have to stroke them."[1]

_____ **Larry Lader to Bernard Nathanson**

How did feminists, especially those in the news media, influence the sexual revolution and the so-called women's liberation movement? How did they collaborate with those who wanted to legalize abortion? How does a revolution occur, anyway, whether political, religious or cultural? There need to be, according to historians, *"an aggrieved class, a climate conducive to radical change, and a weakened government."*[2]

The aggrieved class in the sexual revolution was, of course, women. Part of the revolutionary climate in the sixties was provided by the Vietnam conflict, the undeclared war. The flower children who did the protesting, and those influenced by them, promoted a freer lifestyle that began a movement away from the old guard, away from anything traditional. This atmosphere was supported by antiestablishment sentiments and a quest for liberation, especially for women, that supposedly could be attained by sexual and economic equality, empowerment for the aggrieved class.

The weakened government was the family. Marriage was discouraged, as was the traditional family structure. Flower children asked us all to make love, not war. Not a bad idea. But, the problem was that they weren't talking about true, committed love. They were talking about sex, wherever and whenever possible. They wanted all of the thrills, but none of the responsibility.

Anne Roche Muggeridge describes in her book, *The Desolate City: Revolution in the Catholic Church*,[3] how revolutionaries use these elements to affect changes.

*"They make clear their separation from the old world view, constantly contrasting the bad old ways with the progressive, new ones.*

*Intense propaganda is directed at making the old ideas and disciplines seem outmoded and ridiculous, and the new ones inevitable and irresistible. The interests in grievances of other groups in the society are sympathetically addressed and the advantages of the proposed new order, touted. In this way, key groups in the society are revolutionized. Those who refuse to be co-opted are demoralized by being made to feel that they have been rendered irrelevant by the irresistible."*[4]

The media, then and now, began to chip away at the long-standing societal abhorrence and disdain for abortion. Today, anyone who would have the temerity to say that abortion is wrong, a sin or a crime, is described as old-fashioned and archaic, part of the "religious right." They are painted as unfeeling radicals who want to keep women barefoot and pregnant.

In the mid-nineteenth century, Madame Restell paved the way for today's Yellow Pages' abortion ads, with open advertising for her burgeoning abortion business.

*"Why was there such journalistic unanimity? To judge from the stories, reporters accepted the ideology of both Madame Restell and late 20th century radical feminism. Their stories portrayed abortion as freedom from exploitation, and saw any restrictions on abortion as discrimination against those economically poor."*[5]

Today that same argument is used, repeatedly, by press and politicians, alike. "If poor women can't obtain abortions, they are being discriminated against," and "if the poor continue to breed as they do, we will all suffer."

Alan Guttmacher eventually led the way for Planned Parenthood's agenda by, essentially, using the blueprint for public acceptance of abortion, as described at the 1942 convention of the National Academy of Maternal Health. The arguments for legal abortion were framed as follows: Restrictions against abortion are religious in nature; a woman's privacy must be paramount; an unborn child has no personhood; and, there must be national uniformity in the law.

*"Alan Guttmacher was an active, pro-abortion spokesman and a leading participant in many conferences and convention sessions that provided abortion with an academic cover. Guttmacher's abortion platform was the same as that developed at the Maternal Health conference in 1942: Abortion is liberty, abortion is a woman's right,*

# The Media, Feminism and Abortion

*anti-abortion laws are unfair impositions of biblical morality on others, unborn children are not really human, illegal abortion is unstoppable except by legalization. The difference in the 1950's, however, was that abortionists were successful in targeting three particular groups of leaders: physicians, liberal theologians, and lawyers."* [6]

"To help these groups along, the press "went to bat" for them, took up their cause, promoted their own liberal agenda, and is still doing so today in the name of feminism. The press portrays abortion as freedom from oppression. John Noonan, in his book, "A Private choice: Abortion in America in the Seventies," described how locked into the battle for abortion rights were the media.

"The press was for the abortion liberty. Virtually every major newspaper in the country was on its side, as were the radio stations, the news commentators, the disc jockeys, the pollsters, the syndicated columnists, the editorial writers, the reporters, the news services, the journals of information and the journals of opinion. With the notable exception of three or four syndicated writers...every major molder of public opinion in the press was pro-abortion or indifferent to the issue.

"There was a massive barrier through which any news or opinion contrary to the liberty had to travel. There was not a single large urban newspaper regularly carrying the anti-abortion viewpoint the way Horace Greeley's Tribune had carried the anti-slavery viewpoint."[7]

As in all revolutions, there needs to be an event or a series of events, flags around which to rally. A "flag" was waved in the reporting of the story of Sherri Finkbine, in 1962. She had taken, while pregnant, the drug, thalidomide, as a tranquilizer. The drug that she used was Distaval, which contained thalidomide. Her husband had obtained this drug to use as a sleeping pill, while traveling in Europe. Shortly after taking Distaval, Sherri Finkbine read about thalidomide and its possible effects on developing fetuses, causing them to be missing arms or legs, or parts of their limbs--a condition known as phocomelia (flipperlike limbs). When the connection between these birth defects and the use of thalidomide was discovered, the drug was banned for pregnant women, but those who had already used it had to decide what to do about possible birth defects in their unborn children. Sherri

Finkbine chose abortion. She was a local television actress, who starred in a romper-room type of show in Arizona. She decided to go public with her story..

Her home state of Arizona regularly "got around" the life-of-the-mother requirement for abortion with a panel of physicians who would determine certain abortions as medically necessary. Her abortion was approved just three days after she had first spoken to her doctor. On July 23, 1962, the medical panel had recommended the abortion because there was psychological danger to the mother.

Mrs. Finkbine, however, decided to tell a Phoenix newspaper about her use of thalidomide in order to alert others. Once the story was in the papers, hospital administrators got skittish about an abortion that had already been approved, but didn't want the notoriety that Finkbine's case was causing. They wanted to be certain that the hospital would be perceived as well within its legal bounds. So, they joined the Finkbines in their request for a declaratory judgment saying that her case fit the legal parameters for her abortion, and, thus, free the hospital from any liability. Subsequently, the judge who received the request said that the case was not properly before the court because no one had filed a complaint against the hospital or the Finkbines. This refusal of the judge to hear the case (that wasn't a case at all) was the vehicle, and the press used it for every drop of pro-abortion sympathy they could muster.

Mrs. Finkbine eventually went to Sweden for the abortion. It had been a heyday for the pro-abortion press.

*"Reporters accepted the Finkbine contention that the 'operation' would be performed for the good of the baby. The New York Journal-American quoted Sherri Finkbine as saying, 'We weren't concerned for ourselves but we were concerned for our unborn child. We couldn't, in all conscience, bring into the world a child whose chances seem so utterly hopeless.' Although many people throughout the United States offered to adopt the child if born, the Finkbines were said to be continuing abortion plans for altruistic reasons; a Washington Post reporter told Finkbine of one such offer and noted that she burst into tears saying, 'It doesn't change our minds. It wouldn't be fair to the child.'"[8]*

Certainly, the grief and difficulties for the parents presented by such birth defects is not to be discounted. But, that these abnormalities should be a reason for legal abortion is a giant step into governmental and medical control of decisions about who has (or has not) the potential for a quality life, and who, ultimately, has the right to life. What must handicapped people think when they hear about babies being aborted or left to die because they were less than perfect? If perfection is now the criterion for quality life we are all in trouble. And well we might be with the push for legalization of assisted suicide and euthanasia.

I knew a man who had been born a thalidomide baby. His arms only developed as far as his elbows. I heard him say more than once that he was glad that he had had a chance to live--that his mother had not aborted him. In fact, he was able to eat and drink and do most things by himself--without the use of prostheses. He developed other muscles and motor control, and a good sense of himself and the importance of life. He eventually married and seemed to have as normal a life as the more able of us.

In the specific case of Sherri Finkbine, it had not been widely reported or noted that the studies done on pregnant thalidomide-users had revealed only a twenty percent chance of deformity in their unborn children. It's sad to think that Mrs. Finkbine, over the years, might have wondered about her own child and whether or not he was normal.

During the time the Finkbine story was in the national news, the term, *fetus*, began to be used with great frequency by reporters. The terms, baby or unborn child, were carefully not used. Two things were established for pro-abortion activists with this event: Abortion should be legal and available in the case of fetal anomaly; and the term *fetus* is effective in diverting the public's attention from the humanity of the unborn. Unborn child, pre-born, or baby became "forbidden terminology."

If the Finkbine news story was the simmering of an issue, Norma McCorvey was the boiling point used for the abortion revolution.

> "*Often a revolution simmers before it boils over. When it does the incident that triggers its initial bid for power is often such as would have passed without reaction in an earlier, pre-revolutionary period. Now, when the revolutionaries feel sufficiently strong, the event is represented as being an insult too gross to be borne, the symbol of all the injustice the failing system has ever perpetrated on a helpless society.*"[9]

Norma McCorvey, the Roe of Roe v. Wade was fashioned into that symbol. Not only did she lie about her impregnation by a rapist, but the lie was advanced in order to make a case for all women who are "suppressed and enslaved" by a pregnancy they don't want. Norma was the catalyst for the change that had been brewing. She was used by those more clever than she, and she is still being used. The liberal, feminist media care about her only as long as she is useful. I wonder what they would do if she said she regretted the fact that she sought an abortion and lied. I wonder what they would do if she ever said that she was glad her daughter was born before a legal abortion could take place. Would silence ring through the hallowed halls of media? I think so. I would like to personally meet Norma some day.

Shortly after Roe v. Wade, newspapers gave free publicity to budding abortion clinics. In the San Antonio Light, a wine and cheese fest was promoted for Planned Parenthood, and the Atlanta Journal wrote an article about a "clean facility," giving the address and phone number of the clinic at the end of the article. Not too subtle, I would say.

A few years ago, however, one journalist decided to tell some of the truth of how the abortion question is framed and controlled by the press. David Shaw did a four part series on the press and abortion for the Los Angeles Times.

*"The news media consistently use language and images that frame the entire abortion debate in terms that implicity favor abortion-rights advocates. Abortion-rights advocates are often quoted more frequently and characterized more favorably than are abortion opponents. Events and issues favorable to abortion opponents are sometimes ignored or given minimal attention by the media. Many news organizations have given more prominent play to stories on rallies and electoral and legislative victories by abortion-rights advocates than to stories on rallies and electoral and legislative victories by abortion rights opponents."*[10]

Shaw even criticized his own paper. Indeed, to illustrate the abortion agenda of the *Times*, they had mandated that their reporters never use the term, pro-life or pro-lifers . All references to such activists or activism must be anti-abortion or anti-abortionists. On the other hand, "pro-abortion" and "pro-abortionists," which would be the corresponding and logical, opposite terms, were not to be used. (Note the terms used even in his expose'.) *Abortion-rights activists* is the term still in use, lending it *positivity* and respectability. *Pro-abortionists* doesn't sound so good, does it? Neither does *anti-abortionist*, but it serves a feminist purpose. CNN, (Cable News Network) also has a written directive about which pro-life or pro-abortion words are loaded, and which words can be used by their employees. How can a newspaper or television network justify its demand that their reporters use only their politically-correct terms in order to frame an issue? What about the freedom of the press? Just as it was noted in Nathanson's book, *Aborting America*, Shaw found that:

> *"Abortion opponents are sometimes identified as Catholics (or fundamentalist Christians), even when their religion is not demonstrably relevant to a given story; abortion-rights advocates are rarely identified by religion. Abortion opponents are often described as 'militant' or 'strident'; such characterizations are seldom used to describe abortion-rights advocates, many of whom can also be militant or strident--or both."*[11]

One of the lies about abortion that the media helps promote is that abortions are only performed in the first trimester. Shaw addressed this half-truth in the following paragraph:

> *"But the Supreme Court actually said a woman could have an abortion even in the last three months of pregnancy if that were necessary for 'the preservation of...(her) life or health.' Although only one one-hundredth of 1% of all abortions (about 100 a year) are done after 24 weeks of pregnancy, one-half of 1% (about 8000) are done after 21 weeks and almost 9% (142,000 or almost 400 a day) are done after 12 weeks, according to the Guttmacher Institute."*[12]

The power of the press is awesome. They elect presidents and they bring them down. They can turn on a media darling or they can cover up for him or her. Their reporting of abortionists, for example, who have maimed or killed women in their assembly-line abortion offices, is less than complete. I know of only one investigative report that was done on abortion clinics and doctors. It was published in the Chicago Sun-Times many years ago.
Currently, it is fashionable to be pro-abortion. Conrad, the famous Los Angeles Times cartoonist, at one time was pro-life. His cartoons included an unborn child depicted in his mother's womb with a picket sign saying, "What about my rights, too?" But Mr. Conrad has since changed his style. His pro-abortion cartoons are the norm whenever news events dictate a need for a politically-correct comment. His public advocacy for

abortion is very powerful. I hope his new, more fashionable viewpoint doesn't keep him awake at night.

Six days after Roe v. Wade was handed down, an editorial in the *Orlando Sentinel*, prophetically described our world as it is today. On January 28, 1973, this editorial was published:

> *"The devaluation of morality induced by abortion on demand could, and in all likelihood will, have far reaching effects. Among them are the promotion of promiscuity, depersonalization of the concept of life and activating the destruct button on the family unit as we know it...And what of the woman herself? Abortion by whim could have grave future consequences to her. There is enough unavoidable pain in living without inflicting on oneself, in a period of extremity, the haunting memory of a child that might have been."*[13]

Unfortunately this early, prophetic editorial almost stands alone in its frankness. The press, for the most part became blatantly pro-abortion. In the last twenty years, there has been a concerted effort by politicians and press alike to stifle true "choice." Our rights to exist as a counseling center, as another choice, for example, where we help women so that they can continue their crisis pregnancies, have been so hampered that we cannot even advertise in the Yellow Pages in a competitive manner. We are the only group whose display ads must carry a disclaimer about what we don't offer: "this advertiser does not do abortions or refer for them." A U. S. Representative, Ron Wyden, spearheaded this outrageous, anti-choice legislation, along with a national abortion providers group, the National Abortion Foundation. Our rights to free speech and competition have been blocked at every turn. If a pro-abortion society really believed in "choice," this would not be true. For one thing, we offer full information on abortion, the different types of procedures, and the risks. We cannot stop a woman from making the final decision to abort her child, but if she truly needs to make that decision with full disclosure, then she needs someone other than Planned Parenthood, Family Planning Association, or a professional abortionist to do it.

So, for the abortion revolution we had our events: Norma McCorvey of Roe v. Wade fame, and Sherri Finkbine, who decided she had to "go public" and travel to Europe to secure an abortion that she could have "legally" obtained in Arizona. We had the climate in the sixties: the flower children and their ideas of free love, along with their antiestablishment message. The weakened government needed for a revolution became the family—no longer needed are a married father and mother and their children. Today's family is very complicated, in fact. A woman may have had children by her husband, boyfriends, or a new husband. Children have step-brothers and sisters, half-brothers and sisters, numerous grandparents, or live-in (boyfriend or girlfriend) parents.

Today, sex as entertainment, without consequences, is openly encouraged for women by feminists and the media. Women's magazines, too, reflect this agenda. No longer do *Good Housekeeping* and *Family Circle* set the tone for women.

*Ms. Magazine* and *Cosmopolitan,* for example, present the liberated view. Helen Gurley Brown, *Cosmopolitan*'s Editor-in-Chief, wrote her how-to manual, *Sex and the Single Girl*, at just the right moment, in the mid-sixties. Her book became an overnight sensation--a call to abolish the double standard of chastity for women and promiscuity for men. Her purpose was not to begin holding men responsible for their actions, but, rather, to encourage women to have several sex partners before marriage, sometimes even simultaneously.

Here are some highlights from women's magazines I checked out in April of 1993.

<u>*Cosmopolitan*</u>: This could be called the *Tits*illation magazine. Why women would buy magazines that feature women in various stages of nudity on their covers every month, I don't know. I would prefer Mel Gibson on the cover, fully clothed, myself. I must be in the minority, however. *Cosmopolitan* is still in business. Maybe women believe subliminally that if they buy *Cosmopolitan* they will, vicariously, become as big-breasted and sexy as its cover girls.

Helen Gurley Brown has a regular Editor's column in her magazine. This particular month she talks about several of the issue's articles. She's especially fond of one by a frequent contibutor-writer, Louise Bernikow, who writes about becoming active in the fight against the "increasing erosion of abortion rights." (Abortion on demand for all nine months of the pregnancy isn't enough?)

On page 162, in "The New Activists, Fearless, Funny, Fighting Mad" were the following gems:

*"At Christmastime, Women's Action Coalition carolers stood on the very visible steps of New York City's Saint Patrick's Cathedral, singing 'Rita the red-Nosed Waitress'..."* and *"When pro-choice marches*

were in full swing, women everywhere got up in the morning, called a friend, whipped out a Magic Marker, wrote "U.S. out of My Uterus, Get your nose out of my panty hose and Keep your rosaries off my ovaries on a piece of cardboard and went out to join the crowds. During the Republican convention, protesters paraded in the rudest T-shirt of the year: It showed a woman's shaved pubic area. Read my Lips, it said. No more Bush."[14]

Lovely stuff! Also appearing in Helen's article was an "endearing picture" of Helen with some cats. She loves the picture, she says, that was taken when she was visited by the North Shore Animal League. My title for Helen's piece: "Adopt a Cat--Kill a Baby."

Examples of quotes from two letters to the Advice Column: 1) a sexy voice on the porno calls, "He'd call often, and after I'd bring him to climax, we would discuss all sorts of things." 2) "I'm stuck with my child for the next twenty years, and the prospect is hell."

On the opposite page from the advice column was a very offensive ad of Calvin Klein's with two people copulating on a trapeze!

*Glamour*: The cover story in *Glamour* was "Night and Day. The Double Life of a Topless Dancer." It included a full page photo of the author in her toplessness & G String. She's earning money for college. Really disgusting. Tell me she's liberated and not being used by men (and women). The author was Jenny Silverman. I wonder what her parents think about her full page photo & story. Maybe they should write an article, "My daughter, the Journalist."

There was one reference to marriage and family. On page 100, an ad with a bride & groom for Lane Cedar Chests seemed out of place in this magazine.

On page 56 was an article, "What your Fetus Hears" by an M.D., who discussed studies that had been done on in-utero noise. He said, *"Now that we've found that the womb is a relatively noisy place, we need to think seriously about maternal noise exposure and how it affects an unborn child."* What--a fetus, a non-person, a non-human, hears? This must be doublespeak or doublethink, or maybe it doesn't count because it was such a small article.

The positive side of masturbation was promoted in their Sex & Health feature. One woman said that it helped her when she can't sleep. She wakes up refreshed. Another referring to the risk of AIDS, "I prefer to come home and have sex with myself rather than take the big risk." A truly liberated (lonely) woman!

In "After an Affair:" "Amy had been living with Tim since graduating from college six years earlier and while they often fought, she had always expected that they would be married someday." Not so, however. How tedious of her to think they would be married someday. I thought she was a feminist!

*Good Housekeeping*: Mostly family-oriented; lots of kids and recipes, short stories & articles. Not much of the feminist language or emphasis, as found in the other magazines. Amazing, they still have a market for these subjects!

*McCall's*: There was a good article in this magazine, "Still Single at 38," by an unmarried journalist, who gives a positive viewpoint about not being married--all except her need to tell us she is a practicing heterosexual and how she has to go looking for condoms at three in the morning.

Two family-positive articles about Kevin Costner and Mariel Hemingway, their spouses, and their children appeared in *McCall's*. These famous-celebrity, stable-family stories always seem to be a jinx, however. The famous subjects often get divorced soon after the "everything is perfect" article. I hope that's not true in these cases.

There was a good article on self-esteem for women. A man could easily read it and find worthwhile information for both sexes. That's real feminism: treating men and women as equally human, equally imperfect or vulnerable, and equally as talented and valuable.

*Ms. Magazine*: In an interesting article, "Sexual Harassment: Is There a Feminist Double Standard?," the editors wondered aloud about certain politically-correct silence that had occurred regarding sexual harassment by Senator Bob Packwood, who had been an abortion-rights champion for many years.

*"...In the past, some of us shrugged our shoulders about harassment committed by men we worked with (and even otherwise admired)--to get a bill passed, an amendment stopped, a crucial vote committed. It was a devil's bargain masked as an ethical compromise.*

*Which is why for many women in Oregon and on Capitol Hill, the Washington Post story on Senator Bob Packwood was less a revelation than a confirmation of their own experiences. There had been reasons to keep silent. The senator was a pro-choice vote, when such votes were scarce. For this, NARAL--ignoring many local women's groups that preferred pro-choice challenger Les Au Coin--endorsed*

*Packwood last November.*"[15]

Next to this fairly honest editorial was, however, a short note about lesbian families and how a psychologist "found that offspring of such a family demonstrate a great sense of self-comfort."

Going from magazines to the media giant (television) that has changed our lives forever, it has been noted that American adolescents view nearly 14,000 instances of sexual material on television each year. This was reported in a study conducted by the Center for Population Options in 1991.[16] In the same study, it was found that in all program categories, unmarried heterosexual couples engage in sexual intercourse from four to eight times more frequently than married men and women. My own observations are that in these same programs women seldom get pregnant and both men and women seem to be mysteriously resistant to any strains of sexually transmitted diseases. Would that we could know their secrets!

In action and adventure shows, heterosexual behavior is often associated with violence or a display of power and is rarely depicted in the context of a loving or committed relationship or as an expression of mutual affection.

Results from a survey done in 1987 revealed that afternoon soap operas contained 35 instances of sexual content per hour, or more than one instance every two minutes.

I counseled, over a period of time, a woman who regretted the fact that she had helped her daughter with an abortion some years earlier. Both she and her daughter sought counseling for post-abortion syndrome. Anne told me that one thing she felt had influenced her daughter to have an affair with a married man, and then to have an abortion, was her love of the soap operas. She said that in her daughter's impressionable teen years the sexy love scenes had been her model for love.

Any programs dealing with the abortion issue, whether fiction or non-fiction, often strain to appear as unbiased, but any I have ever viewed have ultimately promoted abortion as the good and proper thing to do.

Feminists and their champions in the press have done women no favors. They have promoted a lie: that abortion is liberating; and, that women should not have to carry "unintended" children to term. They want to indoctrinate our children with sex education in the schools, promote abortion without parental knowledge or consent, and encourage school-based clinics in order to hand out condoms and "safe sex" drivel.

Have the media obscured the truth in order to promote

their feminist and abortion points of view? Unfortunately, yes, and it continues, daily. I saw a bumper sticker not too long ago. It said, "I don't believe the liberal media." I thought it was great! It's nice to know I'm not completely alone.

---

[1] Bernard Nathanson, M.D., *Aborting America*, Doubleday & Company, Inc., Garden City, New York, 1979, p. 50.
[2] Anne Roche Muggeridge, *The Desolate City: Revolution in the Catholic Church*, Harper & Row, 1986, p.50.
[3] Ibid., p. 14.
[4] Ibid.
[5] Marvin Olasky, *The Press and Abortion*, Lawrence Erlbum Assoc., Hillsdale, NJ, 1988, p. 116.
[6] Ibid., p. 85.
[7] John Noonan, *A Private Choice: Abortion in America in the Seventies*, (New York, The Free Press 1979) as quoted in *The Press and Abortion*, Lawrence Erlbum Assoc. Hillsdale, NJ 1988, p. 116.
[8] Marvin Olasky, *The Press and Abortion*, Lawrence Erlbum Assoc. Hillsdale, NJ 1988, pp. 95 & 96.
[9] Anne Roche Muggeridge, *The Desolate City: Revolution in the Catholic Church*, Harper & Row, 1986, pp. 14, 15.
[10] David Shaw, "Abortion Bias Seeps Into News," article in the *Los Angeles Times*, Times-Mirror Corp., July 1, 1990, p. 1.
[11] Ibid., p. 7.
[12] Ibid.
[13] Marvin Olasky, *The Press and Abortion*, Lawrence Erlbum Assoc., Hillsdale, NJ, 1988, pp. 116 & 117.
[14] Louise Bernikow, in "The New Activists: Fearless, Funny, Fighting Mad," *Cosmopolitan Magazine*, April 1993, p. 162.
[15] "Sexual Harassment: Is There a Feminist Double Standard?" *Ms. Magazine*, April 1993, p. 89.
[16] *The Center for Population Options*, August 1991.

# Feminism & The Catholic Church

"...In an age based on the animal philosophy, woman is merely a domestic convenience or a plaything. In an age based on a human philosophy she is man's equal but one who can be taken advantage of or set aside when the need arises. In a supernatural age, one that is imbued with a consciousness of God's part in the world and a conviction of the principles of Christ, woman is a fellow member of the Mystical Body of Christ, an equal before God, a sharer in God's creation."
_____Monsignor Paul J. Hayes[1]

In Monsignor Hayes' book, *The Gifts and Power of Woman*, he describes different ages that are likely to produce different attitudes about women and their places in society and in the church. From his description, I would say that we are in the age based on human philosophy: women have gained more than "plaything" status, but are not viewed as equal members of society or the church. I claim no knowledge of a supernatural age, when it will come or what it will feel like. But where the church is, currently, in its attitudes toward women needs to be re-examined and, possibly, a new direction taken.

Feminists in the church are pushing for ordination of women and for the acquisition of more power in every area, especially in teaching ministries. And priests, bishops and cardinals are stepping back, not sure if these women are right or wrong, or if the traditional church needs to change. They are no longer sure of themselves. Feminist laymen and nuns, however, are very sure of what they want and what they think is needed to gain empowerment for women.

Both the traditional church and the new "feminist" church have important, valid arguments. A change in attitudes about women in the church needs to be examined from both viewpoints. The problem is that right now the vocal feminists, men and women alike, are in the throes of extremism. And the traditional church is not standing strong where it needs to. It's capitulating to those who promote feminist language, for example, in the hope that that's all that's wanted and that those clergy who go along with it will appear liberal and progressive. And feminists who espouse the need for women priests are emphasizing extreme positions, while discarding some of the most basic teachings of their church.

In the supernatural age that Monsignor Hayes speaks of, things would be different. Women would be equal members, brothers, in the body of Christ. Women would be valued members of society and the church, whether married or unmarried. Currently, there is a movement by women members of the church toward empowerment within the structure of the Church. These are active and vocal women who are less concerned about the roles of husbands and wives than they are about the roles of women religious as teachers, theologians, and liturgists. Theirs is a search for superiority and authority, not equality. They are in the convents, teaching in the seminaries, and on college campuses. They have the ears and minds of bishops and cardinals. They are demanding ordination for women and new liturgies designed to rid themselves of patriarchy. They are demanding feminist language that would significantly change prayers, liturgies, music, and even the Bible.

I found a good explanation for the use of feminist language that is now being "strongly recommended" in the Catholic church in a collection of essays about this subject, called, *The Politics of Prayer: Feminist Language and the Worship of God*.[2] The following was written by Michael Levin in his essay, "Linguistics: Use of Generic Man:"

*"Possibly because the only difficulty created by ordinary language is that feminists do not like it, feminist linguistic reform has become a kind of ongoing referendum about feminism itself. In the absence of any clearer purpose, substituting 'person' for 'man' is a concession made to feminists just because feminists demand it. As a result, whatever thought is to be conveyed in the act of communication is consciously subordinated to equity, with the collateral effect of obscuring whatever is actually being said. When clergymen refer to 'Our Father and Mother who are in Heaven', or 'The God of Abraham and Sarah', as many now do, or when contemporary reworkings of the New Testament change the 'Son of God' to 'The human one', they shift attention from religion to the struggle against sexism. Feminist linguistic reform is an*

*attempt to make all thought whatsoever concern feminism to the exclusion of everything else.*"[3]

Donna Steichen reports on the influence of modern feminism in the Catholic Church in her book, *Ungodly Rage.*[4] It is a well-documented report of the movement's agenda and pervasive influence on the Church and society. In the foreword of *Ungodly Rage*, Helen Hull Hitchcock, describes the difference between feminists and traditional women in the Catholic Church, especially relating to the abortion choice.

*"...One thinks, of course, of the open secret that Catholic women are both the leaders and foot soldiers of the anti-abortion movement. Such women are even more victimized by feminists, if possible, than non-feminist men. Women of conviction and action, like the author of this book herself and thousands of other faithful Catholic women--mothers, teachers, religious sisters, professional women, academics and even theologians--who refuse to serve the enraged Goddess of the New Myth and her angry minions, are recognized as a central obstacle, a sign of contradiction, to feminist orthodoxy; and they are treated (or ignored) accordingly. Women who cannot be enlisted in the feminist 'struggle' against the 'patriarchy' are non-persons to feminists. Many Catholic women have experienced this at the 'listening sessions' held in connection with the U.S. bishops' proposed pastoral letter on "women's concerns."*"[5]

Mrs. Steichen describes the last three decades of the development of feminism and its effects on women:

*"Seeing the human failings that follow from original sin but rejecting the doctrine, feminists have blamed them on patriarchy in all its forms, beginning with the Eternal Father. The bitterest irony of this latest battle between the sexes is that it was not men who declared it but feminists. The primary target of secular feminists was the traditional family. Looking back on the cultural expectations prevailing when the sexual revolution began, one can concede that some men demeaned women's characteristic role. Every era has its own imperfections. But it was a far better society for women and children than the present chaotic one, and few women would gladly trade their present state to restore it if*

*they could. The feminists did not call on society to value women's distinctive contributions properly but instead attempted the impossible task of opposing human nature, denying the differences everywhere revealed in experience. Feminists won the battle, and women lost.*

*"More than ever before in the Christian era, women now are expected to submit to sexual exploitation, contraception, abortion, pornography, divorce and permanent assignments in the labor force. Those determined to live as women have traditionally lived often feel they must apologize for, or at least explain, their eccentricity. Single mothers, discarded wives and their children make up the majority of the new poor in this country. A generation of latchkey children is growing up neglected, many of them emotionally and intellectually stunted victims of deficient mothering. At the same time, an indignant masculine backlash against irrational feminist accusations and litigation is emerging to erode further men's protective instincts toward women. Having seen its consequences, most women have abandoned organized feminism, but they still suffer its damaging effects in prevailing sexual permissiveness, employment expectations and marital instability. They are trying to raise their children in their spare time in a culture warped by perverted education, degraded media and widespread doctrinal and moral confusion."*[6]

She certainly doesn't mince words. I spoke to her briefly after a speech that she had given recently. She said that the feminists really do not want to be priests: their purpose is to destroy the traditional, patriarchal church in whatever way that they can. A call for women priests is just a convenient vehicle toward that end. What would Rosemary Ruether, for example, do with the priesthood, if she gained it?

Rosemary Ruether, an ardent feminist, is an extreme example of the enraged woman that Donna Steichen wrote about. Her writings suggest that rather than integration and equality, she desires complete control and change. Ruether aggressively seeks to change the Church, especially. She seeks domination and empowerment, as she criticizes, disdains, and chastises today's Church for its continuing patriarchy.

Ruether is one of the founders of Women-church, supposedly a Catholic women's organization. She advocates a complete displacement of the patriarchy in the Church, a revolution. In order to do this, she has designed some new liturgies that will empower women. From the preface of her book, *Women-Church*[7]:

> *"Women in contemporary churches are suffering from linguistic deprivation and eucharistic famine. They can no longer nurture their souls in alienating words that ignore or systematically deny their existence. They are starved for the words of life or symbolic forms that fully and wholeheartedly affirm their personhood and speak truth about the evils of sexism, and the possibilities of a future beyond patriarchy. They desperately need primary communities that nurture their journey into wholeness, rather than constantly negating and thwarting it. This book takes steps to end that famine of the words of life, and to begin to bake the new bread of life now. We must do more than protest against the old; we must begin to live the new humanity now. We must begin to incarnate the community of faith in the liberation of humanity from patriarchy in words and deed, in new words, new prayers, new symbols and new praxis. This means that we need to form gather communities to support us as we set out on our exodus from patriarchy."*[8]

Feminism, in an even more bizarre form, can be found in the writings of Starhawk (Miriam Simos Rahsman). She has a formula for a new religious ritual designed for her followers of witchcraft:

> *"...the form of ritual is circular: We face each other, not an altar or a podium or a sacred shrine, because it is in each other that the Goddess is found. Every Witch is Priestess or Priest: there are no hierophants, no messiahs, no avatars, no gurus. The Goddess says, 'If that which you seek, you find not within yourself, you will never find it without. For I have been with you from the beginning.'"*[9]

Somewhere in the middle of this vast expanse of differences between Rosemary Reuther, Starhawk and Donna Steichen, we find Denise Lardner Carmody. She is an ex-nun, who married an ex-priest. She actively promotes the ordination of women to the priesthood, but, more conservatively, remains pro-life. In her book, *Double Cross*,[10] Carmody suggests adoption

# Feminism & the Catholic Church

as an alternative to abortion:

> "However, only the hopelessly naive would think that even a thousandfold improvement in our attitudes and practices would eliminate unwanted pregnancies. For the vast majority of these pregnancies the solution which is most rational and consistent with the ethical viewpoint I have been developing is adoption. If the fetus is innocent humanity with the right to life, then this woman, and the father of her child, and representatives of society at large ought to arrange for the child's being raised in other circumstances. At present we assume many of the arguments of the anti-abortion position and make adoption much more difficult than it should be.
>
> "I am not referring to the regulations that are designed to insure the child's welfare in an adoptive home. I am referring to the attitude that a child is only its parents' responsibility, and to the refinement of this attitude: the feeling that the pregnant woman got herself with child and that consequently the child is only her burden. One might be able to mount a defense of this position--I think it would be feeble-were there no appropriate people longing to adopt children. But in fact the mismatch between the huge number of fetuses being killed each year and the huge number of people wanting to adopt children is another sign of the dysfunction of our social systems. Just as the mismatch between the people going hungry in our society and the food being wasted shouts that we have an absurd system, so does the mismatch between abortion and the desire to adopt. The privacy of the adoption decision, as defined by the current law once again flies in the face of the overall social reality and the overall common good."[11]

Her steadfast belief in the pro-life viewpoint, along with her untraditional support for women priests, must be a difficult line to follow with friends and enemies alike.

Judith Wilt, on the other hand, calls herself a feminist and a Catholic. I doubt the Catholic part. In her book, *Abortion, Choice & Contemporary Fiction*,[12] she seems desperately to be seeking to make a pro-abortion view acceptable to herself and to others. She strains to claim religiosity:

> *"As a feminist and a Catholic, I believe a woman's freedom to abort a fetus is a monstrous, a tyrannous, but a <u>necessary</u> freedom in a fallen world."*[13] (emphasis in the original, but I would have italicized this lie, anyway)

She continues, later:

> *"The pro-life worldview, like Lacan's imaginary, is immersed in, and at home with, transcendence, confident that all the 'surprises' of human experience have a grace in them; that all new directions, even those that hit with the force of a blow, are one direction; that the plenteous self, the oceanic unity in the mirror, will be reached in the post-mortal end. The pro-choice worldview, bereft or uncertain of this end, dwells in Lacan's symbolic order, ready to speak, ready to plan, ready for the long, complex arc of reasoned thought toward best possible choice."*[14]

In other words, women who are submissive to a Divine will, submissive to what life brings them, accepting trials (and unexpected children) are naive and simplistic. And those, who are thinking, intellectually-correct individuals understand that as long as they employ reasoned thought, whatever their decision, it is the correct one. As Mary Hunt of Catholics for A Free Choice strained to do on the talk-radio program, so does Wilt strain to make acceptable the choice of abortion by contrasting the pro-life vs. pro-choice viewpoints as either naive, simple-minded (the pro-life view) or intellectual and logical (the pro-abortion view).

Feminists, rather than moving toward or convincing the church and society, in general, that women possess worthwhile qualities and abilities that should be honored and recognized equally, instead want to empower themselves, seek to dominate (the very thing that angers them about the patriarchy).

Where do I, personally, stand in all of this? Somewhere in the middle, I suspect. I don't feel that women need to be or should be priests. But, I long for intellectual and spiritual recognition of women's abilities, of their equal needs and rights within their own families and within the Church family. Yes, man should be the head of his family, as long as he merits that role, and as long as he loves his wife and children, with all that that includes. But, if he sees his role as authoritarian only, or if he abuses his family, either psychologically or physically, he should lose his right of leadership.

And, the Church's bishops and priests should recognize the gifts that women can give to the Church. At this point in time, only the vocal radicals are getting their message through. This has resulted in feminist activism that seems to undermine our future priests in the seminaries, our current priests in their parishes, and our laymen in liturgical committees. True equality for women will not be attained by gaining the nonsensical, clumsy use of feminist language in the newer versions of scripture, nor by eventually ordaining women priests. It will be attained when men and women listen to one another, and act from a truly Christian, truly spiritual perspective--when both men and women understand what St. Paul meant by submission and love. They are interchangeable, movable qualities that should pervade all interactions between men and women, and women and their Church.

At the time of Christ's life on earth, women in Jewish society were not granted many rights, were not even considered part of the political or religious communities. Indeed, even the count of five thousand people described in the loaves and fishes' passage in the Bible was probably not accurate because women and children were not counted at that time--only men were. It does seem, however, from the New Testament account of Jesus' life that He honored, revered, and respected women. Every time women were present with Jesus, He spoke to them, included them and demonstrated a great love for them.

St. Paul, on the surface at least, does not seem to share this attitude. The following has always been difficult for me to understand:

*"Wives should be submissive to their husbands as if to the Lord because the husband is head of his wife just as Christ is head of his body the church, as well as its savior....Husbands, love your wives, as Christ loved the church. He gave himself up for her to make her holy....Husbands should love their wives as they do their own bodies....No one ever hates his own flesh; no, he nourishes it and takes care of it as Christ cares for the church, for we are members of his body." (Saint Paul*

*to the Ephesians 5:22.)*

Must I be submissive in all things? Does my husband really rule, with all the authority of a king? What if my ideas are better? What if he is bad-tempered, a drunk? What if he abuses me? What if circumstances are such that I must take over for a time, or press my point because of a conviction that I am right and he is wrong about a serious decision?

In his book, *The Gifts & Power of Woman*, Monsignor Hayes explains this difficult passage, in part through the eyes of love and all that love means.

*"True, Paul speaks of the husband's place as the head, but it is not a place of control and demanded obedience. Read further, and the obligations of a husband inspire a sense of awe. He must have a sacrificial love. He must love his wife as Christ loves the Church. In other words he must give his entire life for her.* "[15]

Husbands should love their wives as they love their own bodies: what a description of a lifelong giving of oneself--to love their wives as their own bodies. This is such a powerful statement--the one I never seemed to get to when I would read this passage. All I saw was "red," when I got to the words, "be submissive," and I never seemed to get beyond that. Unfortunately, I don't know if men ever get farther in the reading of that passage, either. Certainly, I haven't seen examples of men loving their wives or girlfriends as their own flesh, in my experience with women and their problem pregnancies. If they did, they wouldn't pressure them to get abortions.

As I mentioned earlier in this chapter, it is now "strongly recommended" that the reading used on Holy Family Sunday in the Catholic church, St. Paul's call for wives to be submissive, be deleted and a shorter version of this Bible passage read. I, who just a few short years ago choked on this passage and teased my husband that I would delete the submissive part the next time I was a lector, now prefer that the entire passage be read.

A lot of the controversy about submission was explained very well in an encyclical on Christian Marriage, written by Pope Pius XI.

*"Subjection does not deny or take away the liberty which fully belongs to the woman both in view of her dignity as a human person, and in view of her most noble office as wife and mother, nor does it bid her obey her husband's every request if not in harmony with right reason or with the dignity due to the wife...But it forbids that exaggerated liberty which cares not for the good of the family.....If the man is the head, the woman is the heart, and as he occupies the chief place in ruling, so she may and ought to claim for herself the chief place in love."*[16]

There is a time for submission, for both sexes, and a time for love, whether it is shown in compassion, understanding, and sensitivity to one another, or when it is shown by a man or a woman who stands firmly committed to what is right for their relationship. Love and submission are needed from both partners, and both need to be respected for their ideas and needs.

Will there be women priests? Will this radically change the face of the Catholic Church? Or will the revolution accomplish equality and respect for women within its present, traditional framework? Will this satisfy the current, vocal feminist? Or will there be a split? Will we eventually have an American Catholic Church and a Roman Catholic Church? Will feminists really change the Bible to exclude most male references?

I don't have the answers, but I do know that ideas and events surrounding these issues will continue to be very turbulent going into the twenty-first century. My hope is that all of us, men and women alike, will learn to appreciate and respect one another as equals. My prayer is that the supernatural age that Monsignor Hayes describes will be a reality, and that women will move forward, coming from a place of strength, equality, and from a truly God-centered perspective.

---

[1] Msgr. Paul J. Hayes, *The Gifts & Power of Women*, Daughters of St. Paul, Boston, 1987, p. 43.

[2] *The Politics of Prayer, Feminist Language in the Worship of God*, Edited by Helen Hull Hitchcock, Ignatius Press, San Francisco, 1992.

[3] Michael Levin, "Linguistics: Use of Generic Man," Ibid., p. 121.
[4] Donna Steichen, *Ungodly Rage*, Ignatius Press, San Fracisco, 1991.
[5] Helen Hull Hitchcock, Ibid., p. iv.
[6] Donna Steichen, Ibid., p. 379.
[7] Rosemary Ruether, *Women-church*, Harper & Row, San Francisco, 1985, pp. 4 &5.
[8] Ibid.
[9] Starhawk, *Spiral Dance: A Rebirth of the Ancient Religion of the Great Goddess*, SF/Harper & Row, 1979, pp. 197 & 198.
[10] Denise Lardner Carmody, *Double Cross*, Crossroad, NY, 1986, p. 119.
[11] Ibid.
[12] Judith Wilt, *Abortion, Choice & Contemporary Fiction*, University of Chicago Press, Chicago & London, 1990, pp. 6 & 7.
[13] Ibid.,xii.
[14] Ibid., pp. 6 & 7.
[15] Msgr. Paul J Hayes, *The Gifts & Power of Women*, Daughters of St. Paul, Boston, 1987, p. 62.
[16] Pope Pius XI, from "Encyclical on Christian Marriage," in *The Gifts & Power of Women*, Daughters of St. Paul, Boston, 1987, p. 49.

# Dear Ms. Chairperson

> "The strategy of marketing abortion rights under the label of 'pro-choice' was conceived by a 'Madison Avenue' advertising agency. And it was a clever one. After all, the word 'choice' strikes at the very heart of what we as Americans hold most dear."[1]
> _____Dayton Right to Life Society

One of the feminist agenda items has been to change our language, to either dilute gender distinction or to replace, whenever possible, the word, *man*, with person. Language is very powerful, and, indeed, much of the feminist agenda has been advanced by these changes. I find the word, *chairperson*, for example, silly and clumsy. I am insulted by it. I always considered myself to be part of the family of man. I was always happy to be a chairman or be part of a group headed by a female chairman. *Spokesperson* is clumsy, too. I was recently the foreperson on a jury. I consistently referred to myself as the foreman and signed as such. I often wondered what the judge, a woman, thought of my little acts of rebellion. Should she have been a judgeperson?

Ms. has never done much for me, either. I guess it's supposed to hide the fact of my marital status--make me sort of a generic woman. I don't believe that my worth or personality should be defined by my marital status and the fact that every woman becomes a generic Ms. doesn't give us any additional power or respect, that I can see.

I, myself, am content with no title at all. When I get mail from all of the really important organizations, like The Publishers Clearing House, where I most likely will win a million dollars, they address me by my first name, in bold letters, printed in by a "personal" computer. Why shouldn't my friends do the same? Who needs Ms., Mrs. or Miss? I don't. Now, if I were a doctor, *Dr.* might be nice, and if I were a priest or minister, *Father* or *Reverend* might also be nice. But Ms.--how does that define or honor me? What does it do for me?

On the other hand, the new way of referring to women in news articles is to use their last names only, as in, "Hamilton said she didn't rob the convenience store." I guess this is supposed to connote my equality with men, as in, "Smith said he didn't rape Jones." I think I would prefer Gail or Mrs. Hamilton or Miss Hamilton or even Ms. Hamilton, in that case. It seems to me that if I were simply *Hamilton* I might be judged more harshly, whereas with Ms. or Mrs. Hamilton I might get off with probation.

The use of the word, *patriarchy*, usually sounds pretty bad, whenever it's used--calling to mind threatening images of men sitting on thrones or cracking whips. It implies that one group (men) have unlimited power over another group (women). I kind of like men myself, even though I don't want them to have any unequal or unjustified power over me. Patriarchy implies that all men are mean, ugly slave masters. It just isn't so, however.

When women discuss or write about a patriarchy, it is usually a call to arms, a call to strive for empowerment. They seem to be saying that they want to overthrow the existing government, the patriarchal social order! I don't like living in a patriarchy, either. But would a matriarchy be any better? Wouldn't an equal and shared social order be preferable? Is it possible?

Even though we hear a lot about feminism these days, the term, *women's liberation*, isn't used much anymore. It was overdone for a long time, eventually becoming a pejorative term that conjures up images of women in the sixties who burned their bras and walked around topless (with flowers in other places.) If *women's lib* is dead, what terms have replaced it? We now have a new vocabulary of feminist language. Some words, like the gender-neutral ones noted above, are subtle. Some are not so subtle.

Goddess is being used quite liberally, at the moment. Women, and some men, are referring to God, as "God, she said," and "God, she would."

Currently, in the church's need for change, some of the language in the songs we sing has been changed. "Good Will to

# Dear Ms. Chairperson

Men" at Christmastime is now "Good will to all." "Good Christian Men, Rejoice" is now "Good Christians, All, Rejoice."

I used to feel a kinship with all of my fellow human beings. I like both men and women. But, ladies, don't you think that *Ms., chairperson, spokesperson*, etc. is just a joke on us? I see men snickering behind their dinner menus. I hear them whispering, "Give them Ms., give them chairperson--we're still in charge." Rather than discussing the seriousness of equality, dignity, and respect for women, they give us these concessions.

Other words have had their meanings changed in order to gain the advantage or obscure the truth in the abortion debate. The word, *choice*, has become the most ill-used word in modern America's vocabulary. When those who are pro-abortion speak on the subject of choice they never finish the sentence. They say, "I am pro-choice," supposedly painting themselves as open and compassionate. If they were to finish the sentence they would have to say, "I am pro-choice about abortion." And, if pressed to fully define their declaration of a pro-choice stand, they would have to say, "I support a woman's right to kill her unborn child." But they won't truthfully and openly make such statements. They talk about *fetuses, products of conception and procedures*, obscuring the truth in order to appear to have the moral high ground.

Language is very powerful. It can subtly change cultural standards and it can boldly change ideas and ways of relating to one another. We need to face reality about the liberation of women, about abortion, and about the relationships between men, women, and their children. And, we need to use terms that are honest, not euphemisms made up by Madison Avenue in order to conceal the truth.

A real *coup* in clever labeling is *Planned Parenthood*. Their purpose is to discourage parenthood, not promote it. And, the results of their ideology and agenda have been disastrous, a failure. For one thing, Planned Parenthood has not decreased teen pregnancy; in fact, it has increased dramatically since they have become so influential in our schools. They have promoted promiscuity, teen abortions, and general moral confusion because their basic philosophy is that teens are young animals who can't possibly be intelligent enough to control themselves.

Planned Parenthood offers many services related to human sexuality. In their main brochure, PPLA (Planned Parenthood, Los Angeles) says that they will provide for teens, with no questions asked and no parental involvement, the following services and items: Abortion, up to 22 weeks; the Pill, diaphragm, IUD, foam and condoms, Norplant, cervical caps, sponges, and natural family planning. (I question this one and how often it is offered.) Abortion to 22 weeks for teen girls??!!

I recently spoke to a 14-year-old girl who was 15 weeks pregnant. She told me that she was going to be transported from a Family Planning Associates clinic to a downtown facility (where they do late-term abortions). She said that no one knew about the pregnancy or the abortion, set for that day. Think about it! Beside this little girl, only the clinic staff and I knew about this traumatic, possibly dangerous procedure that she was submitting herself to. If there were complications, who would help her?

Planned Parenthood tells us in their brochure that they are advocates in the fight for abortion rights. The most obvious euphemism is, of course, their name. It should read Nonparenthood. They really do not promote parenting. Surprise, surprise!

<u>Planned Parenthood is the largest provider of abortion in this country.</u> And, they receive *beaucoup* government dollars to further this insanity. They will tell you, of course, that the federal funds are used only for education. I, for one, would like to see their books. And, of course, funds that are provided by the government for education free up funds used for their aggressive abortion/condom/pill agenda.

I interviewed a friend of a friend, who is a Counselor for Planned Parenthood in the Midwest. I decided to print the telephone interview as it unfolded, without embellishment. But I

# Dear Ms. Chairperson

take the writer's privilege of analyzing and arguing with the counselor after the fact, so to speak, because I had promised my California friend that the interview would not be a debate.

**What is your title at Planned Parenthood? Is this a full-time position? What are your duties?**

*"I am a Full-time supervisor at the Teen Services Center. I have a B.A. in Psychology, working on my Masters in Health Education."*

**What, in your own words, is the mission statement of PP?**

*"In general, to provide services and education to increase and control fertility."*

**What prompted you to become active and to work for PP?**

*"Initially, I saw the need for education and a change of attitude in the area of birth control and my wanting to help do this."*

**I'd like to read from an interview I had this morning with a 33-year-old woman, who has had a sexually promiscuous lifestyle. Would you please comment on her story? (I read Deana's story, who did identify feminism and the sixties' sexual revolution as the main motivations for her regrettable lifestyle that led to promiscuity, one tubal pregnancy, contraction of the human papilloma virus (HPV), cervical cancer, and infertility.)**

*"I haven't personally been involved with the feminist movement."*

(My *after-comment*: She was unwilling to express a view on any of the details of the woman's story, including her fight for life with cervical cancer, her inability to conceive a child, after having one tubal pregnancy, or her ongoing battle with the Human Papilloma virus.)

**What is your personal feeling about abortion?**

*"It needs to be an individual's right to choose what she wants to do. There should be a right to have an abortion."*

(My comments: Here again, she wasn't willing to speak very personally about abortion. It seemed that she was just repeating PP's politically-correct answer about *choice*.)

**How do you feel about the PP statement?: "Parental involvement laws in general cause teenagers to delay an abortion, either by creating a longer decision-making process, by involving them in conflict with their parents, or by forcing them to go through an often lengthy judicial process. Later abortions cost more and**

involve greater risks to a girl's health than early abortions.?"

"*I agree with the statement. The girls have a major decision to make at a difficult time. The clinics will really try to counsel girls.*"

(My comments. Who owns our children? How can parental rights regarding the physical and emotional care of our children be swept away by an organization and a government who think they know better than we do? How dare they take my rights and my children from me?! )

**What about complications? Shouldn't the parents know ahead of time? What about serious situations, like hemorrhaging or a perforated uterus, that would necessitate a girl being taken to the hospital?**

"*Our doctors have gone in to help girls with complications on off-hours, even.*"

(My comment: The doctors will go in *at all hours* in order to avoid any young woman or teen having to go to the hospital, where she would have to tell where she obtained the abortion that has caused her to hemorrhage or where she developed an infection, or worse. We get calls from women with physical complications one or two days after an abortion quite regularly.)

**What would you tell your teenage daughter to do if she were wanting to be sexually involved with a young man or if she is pregnant? (Note: my interviewee is a young, married woman who does not have children at this time.)**

"*I would tell her to wait until she is in a meaningful relationship. If she were pregnant I wouldn't pressure her one way or the other.*"

(All I can say is, "Wait until this Planned Parenthood Counselor has children. Either she will change her mind (about 180 degrees, hopefully) or she will stand by this philosophy and her teen children will not find the moral guidance or help they need from Mom and Dad." I sincerely hope she will change her mind.)

**Do you consider yourself a feminist?**

"*I wouldn't consider myself an activist, but I have noticed that at work there is still more inequality than there should be.*""

**Do you have any additional comments?**

# Dear Ms. Chairperson

> *"After having worked with teens for so long, I wish the parents would talk more to their kids about sex."*

(I have to agree with her, but I must add that I wish Planned Parenthood wouldn't talk to them at all, because they don't really have my children's welfare in mind or in their plan.)

**How do you view the work that I do, which is essentially offering help to those who might otherwise feel they had no choice but abortion?**

> *"I think the alternatives <u>and</u> abortion should be presented in an unbiased way."*

Instead of my "after-comments" about her final statement, I would like to offer a comment by Dr. George Flesh, the obstetrician who used to perform abortions, but changed his mind:

> *"I believe that tearing a developed fetus apart, limb by limb, simply at the mother's request is an act of depravity that society should not permit. We cannot afford such a devaluation of human life, nor the desensitization of medical personnel that it requires. This is not based on what the fetus might feel, but on what we should feel in watching an exquisite, partly formed human being dismembered, whether one believes that man is created in God's image or not."*[2]

In 1993, Planned Parenthood decided that because there was a dwindling number of doctors who would perform abortions, they would start a 3-year, $1.5 million program to do abortions.

My question is, "If Planned Parenthood values *choice* so much for the individual, why don't they value choice for society as a whole?" It would seem to me that if more and more doctors are unwilling to perform abortions, a natural choice has been made. Their anxiety about fewer doctors performing abortions is because they are, in truth, pro-active, not neutral, on the abortion issue.

If there weren't enough doctors to do such grisly deeds on a regular basis, then eventually more and more women might have to wait a day or so when they are considering abortions. And, if they wait a day or so they might change their minds. If they change their minds once, they might not have any abortions, ever. Then, if they have no abortions because they have experienced what it means to be pregnant and have a child, the whole theory of abortion solving women's problems might be seriously damaged. And, the propaganda that abortion is a moral good and an answer to women's crisis pregnancies might be seen for the lie that it is.

Who profits from an abortion? Planned Parenthood, abortionists, fathers of the unborn who "get out of town," as quickly as possible, and parents of teens who don't want to deal with a sticky problem. Who are the victims? The pregnant women who have to deal with it for the rest of their lives, and the unborn children, of course, who have no *choice*.

One of the cases that I did not deal with directly, but had direct knowledge of, was the experience of a young woman and her boyfriend who did not want an abortion. But her parents did. They spirited their daughter away to a hotel room when they couldn't keep the young couple apart. She was kept incommunicado for several days. Her boyfriend called the Right to Life League, and a search was implemented for his pregnant girlfriend. She was finally found, dramatically, as she was being prepared for the abortion she did not want. She was actually up on the table as her boyfriend found her. She cried with relief when she saw him. They got married and had their baby, together. Are they living happily ever after? Last I heard, they are. Would they be if the grandparents had had their way? Certainly, no one is guaranteed everlasting bliss, but if the girl's parents had forced her to have the abortion, many lives and relationships would have been broken.

In what I consider a real slip about true, informed choice, Planned Parenthood of Los Angeles (PPLA) uses in a handout the following:

*"Requiring even 24 hours, however, could result in a much longer delay, or prevent the abortion altogether, because: 83% of U.S. Counties have no abortion providers, so that many women have to travel some distance for services. Often, public transportation is unavailable.*

# Dear Ms. Chairperson

*Most clinics do not have daily services; in some cases a woman may have to wait several days for the next opportunity, an especially serious obstacle if she has had to travel.*"[3]

    PLLLLeeeasse, I can't believe that a life-changing, serious decision can't wait 24 hours. We're not talking about waiting to have an eyeglass prescription filled! I know of cases where laminaria have been inserted for a mid-term abortion and less than 24 hours later (the usual waiting time for the laminaria to stretch the cervix and bring on labor) the woman has changed her mind about having the abortion! The real reason Planned Parenthood wants women to get in for an abortion immediately is because otherwise they might have second thoughts.

    Also included in this particular handout is the information that when Minnesota enacted stricter abortion laws, including parental consent, the teen birth rate rose 38%. What this statement didn't tell you is that <u>the teen pregnancy rate decreased dramatically at the same time</u>. So, if 38% more of the teens who got pregnant chose life for their babies instead of abortion--and more teens did not get pregnant, we've got a large percentage of Minnesota's teen girls who remained whole--unscarred and unwounded from either of these traumatic experiences.

    What happened when abortion became legal? The back-alley abortionists moved to the front office, that's what happened. To say abortion is safe because it is legal is a lie. Abortion destroys human beings, women's emotional lives and often their ability to have subsequent children, families, and relationships.

    So, Ms. Chairperson, before you consider your choice to be a completely independent, sexually-liberated individual, consider all of the facts; look beyond the euphemisms and decide how to be in charge of your life. No matter how many slogans, like *safe sex, freedom of choice*, or a *woman's right to choose* are forced into your subconscious, the truth about contraceptives or the immorality and traumatic effects of abortion don't change.

A woman's choice whether or not to risk becoming pregnant began when she decided to engage in a sexual relationship, whether that relationship is two years, two days, or even two hours long! Years ago, early in the abortion controversy, I listened to a call-in radio show. The discussion was abortion, and I just had to give my opinion. The host asked, after I had made some obviously pro-life comments, *"You mean, when somebody has just been a little naughty, they should be made to pay for this mistake by continuing an unwanted pregnancy?"* A *little naughty* was such a deprecating phrase intending to indicate that the subject was of little importance. How far he was from the truth about humans, their choices and consequences. An unwanted pregnancy involves three human beings and decisions about life and death, no matter what word games are used. An unborn human being has intrinsic value; it is not a trivial consequence of someone's being naughty.

The abortion industry seems to require a new language. *Choice* is the big word. Some of the other "meaningful" words to watch for are: *Products of Conception, Procedure, Termination, Fetus, Reproductive Freedom.*

A telephone conversation, when calling an abortion clinic, might sound like this: *"Are you seeking a termination? When can we make an appointment for the procedure? Your reproductive freedom means that you can expel the fetus at 8:00 AM on Saturday. The products of conception will be removed by a suction abortion. Please have your procedure fee ready, in hand, in cash, when you come in."*

If the *uneuphemized* version of this telephone conversation were used, it would be an entirely different story: *"Do you want an abortion? When can we make an appointment for the extraction of your unborn child? His body will be removed by a suction machine, something like a high-powered vacuum cleaner. Of course, he will look like a blob of tissue <u>after</u> this happens. Please have your cash ready when you come in-- we have a tight schedule to keep, and your cash ensures that there will be no record of this procedure."*

*Termination* and *procedure* both are used instead of the word, abortion. *Reproductive freedom* refers to a woman's legal right to abort her unborn child. Fetus, in Latin, means young one,

# Dear Ms. Chairperson

and is useful because one doesn't have to say baby or unborn child. It's clinical. *Expel* is usually used when a description of abortion is needed. The most common *expulsion* (before thirteen weeks) is by vacuum aspiration (suction abortion). The *products of conception* are used instead of *the baby*, after he has been ripped from his mother's womb. *Procedure* fees equal the cost of one human life, some cost less and some cost more. It depends on the neighborhood and the overhead.

I am frankly afraid for my children, their friends, and my future grandchildren. Planned Parenthood, the National Education Association, and drug companies who *donate* to school clinics would like nothing better than to indoctrinate our children from toddler through their adulthood. In fact, they are able to do this quite freely already. The push for government day care, the campaign against a school voucher system, and the establishment of school-based clinics all work together to deprive parents of their natural rights.

"No more lies, no more euphemisms" would be a better slogan for our young women (and young men). It would be a good start on the road to real freedom, real empowerment and a new feminism that lifts up, rather than destroys.

Language is very powerful. It can change hearts and minds. It can create a whole new mindset. But the effects of this so-called sexual revolution and so-called freedom for women have been devastating. The equality and justice that are supposedly the goals, the need to empower one's sisters by bringing down the patriarchy, and the happiness that is supposed to come from all of this have brought the American woman and the American family into a position of weakness, disarray, dysfunction, and general confusion. Our children are no longer valued or respected. And, neither are the women who abort them. Abortion is big business--no matter what euphemisms are used.

Ms. Chairperson needs to get her act together. She needs to see and believe in her own intrinsic worth, without need of approval or stability from a father, a boyfriend or a husband. She needs to be able to live and prosper on her own, undamaged by a promiscuous lifestyle, sexually-transmitted disease, or an abortion experience. It's true that this will take some degree of self-control, self-respect, and self-esteem on her part, but it will all be worth it in the end. At this point in time, everything is working against her: her parents' unstable marriages; her divorced parents' lifestyles (their girlfriends and boyfriends living in); her schools who give her no direction, but a values-free sex education; Planned Parenthood, who recruits her into a philosophy that is self-destructive; and the feminists who tell her her worth is dependent upon her *freedom* to do whatever she wants.

We need to use language to tell the truth, not to propagandize by calling a thing something that it isn't. The *choice* to kill or not to kill, is nothing more than license. *Products of conception* are really pre-born babies, and Ms. Chairperson is still a woman, one of the two sexes, and a part of *man*kind, no matter how she is addressed.

Real choice is the great American dream. The liberties and life options that we enjoy with our form of government, are unequaled in history. Choice is good; choice is essential. But selfish, destructive options, without limits, as in the choice to have an abortion, will eventually destroy our great dream, our treasured freedoms.

---

[1] *Just the Facts* brochure, distributed by Dayton Right to Life Society, 1990.
[2] George Flesh, M.D., "Why I No Longer Do Abortions," Los Angeles Times, Sept. 12, 1991.
[3] "Teenage Women, Abortion, and the Law," *Fact Sheet*, National Abortion Federation, August 1990.

# Abortion & Religion

"The charge of 'imposing morality' reflects confusion about the relationship of law and morality. All laws, insofar as they reflect a community's sense of fairness and justice, necessarily have a moral component. To remove this moral component would make law an arbitrary instrument for the control of the weak by the more powerful elements of society."[1]       John Jefferson Davis

The observance of morality does not mean that we as a society are sanctioning a specific dogma or religious doctrine. Certainly, man is distinguished from the rest of nature, from the law of the jungle, by his understanding of morals and principles, his conscience. This does not necessarily demonstrate that his ethical judgments or actions are a teaching of any one particular church.

The right to life for all humans, from conception to natural death, is not a religious issue, as some have tried to frame it. It's an issue of basic human rights--of morality vs. expediency.

Dr. Bernard Nathanson, in his book, *Aborting America*, describes several strategy meetings in which Lawrence Lader, a fellow abortion activist, proposed ways to present the Catholic Church as the chief opponent of abortion, and to present its hierarchy in a very unflattering light. Lader was clever. He said he didn't want to broadbrush all Catholics. In fact, he wanted to recruit liberal Catholics to the abortion cause.

*"For their part, of course, the Catholic bishops were to play right into our hands, by their heavy-handed politicking, making abortion appear to be purely a 'Catholic issue' rather than an interreligious one."*[2]

The fact that Christians, especially Roman Catholic Christians, are involved and sometimes take the lead in pro-life activities is true, but the National Abortion Rights Action League (NARAL) and the media are inaccurate in their portrayal of strong, organized, religious involvement. If it were more organized and united, a lot more would be accomplished.

The interesting thing about all of this anti-Catholic, anti-abortion rhetoric is the fact that neither historically, nor presently, were the clergy in the forefront of promoting the pro-life message. Again, from the book *Aborting America*,:

> "The U.S. statutes against abortion have a non-sectarian history. They were put on the books when Catholics were a politically insignificant minority. James C. Mohr's important historical study *Abortion in America : The Origins and Evolution of National Policy, 1800-1900 91(1978)* proves conclusively that even the Protestant clergy was not a major factor in these laws. Rather the laws were an achievement of the American Medical Association and the 'regular physicians, who were combatting fly-by-night medical practice.'"[3]

Who, then, really, are the activists in the pro-life movement?

I attended my first meeting of the Valley Chapter of the Right to Life League in February of 1970. I remember the month and year well. I was a new Mom. At this point in my life, I still do not know why I responded to a small ad in my church bulletin (placed there by a fellow member of the church, not the pastor) about an organizing meeting for a "right to life" organization. Why would anyone with a 7-week-old baby want to get involved in something as emotional and time-consuming as organizing a group for social activism? I was ignorant on the subject of legal abortion and totally inexperienced about the commitment involved in activism of any kind. But, I had just experienced a dramatic change in my world view that occurred the minute I delivered my firstborn child, Christine. So, my sudden awakening to a world outside of my own narrow, personal one led me into the abortion debate and the eventual activism that came with it.

A few months after that first meeting, I saw on the evening news, a suction abortion--as I held my new little daughter in my arms. I have never forgotten the tears rolling down my face, as I realized that I was watching a girl or boy's life being destroyed, being sucked out of its mother, as I nursed my own precious child.  How could they put this on the nightly news?

I remember having that same feeling of helplessness and shock when I "eyewitnessed," via the 6:00 o'clock news, a reporter being gunned down in Nicaragua at the height of their civil war.  That evening all of the news stations showed the particularly grisly sight of a man buckling from a bullet to his chest, struggling to get up, and being shot several more times, over and over and over again.

"Hey, I wanted to say each time, "there are 'live' people there!  There is a pre-born human being in that woman's womb.  That reporter in Nicaragua wasn't hurting anyone, why shoot him?  Why doesn't someone help them?  Why doesn't someone stop this violence?  This is happening now!  Why doesn't someone stop this abortion, this murder?"

Some of us did decide to try to stop this terrible thing.  Some had reasons similar to mine for becoming involved.  They cared about the unborn children and they cared about our country.  Some had been touched personally by an illegal or legal abortion.  Some had handicapped children they loved, even though there were difficulties in their lives.  Some had large families and were glad to say that they valued each child, even though they always struggled financially.  Some had only one child or no children.  Some were adoptive parents, who were grateful that a young woman had had the courage to give her child to them to love and raise.  We were all different and we were all coming together, trying to organize some kind of educational campaign against what we believed to be the coming horror of abortion on demand.

Our first plan was to go to the churches, asking for their help, so that we could reach their congregations with the pro-life message.  What happened then still saddens me.

We decided to contact pastors of all faiths, individually, by making appointments with them, telling them what we knew about legal abortion, where we felt the trend was heading, and asking if we could speak to their congregations. I will always remember visiting several Protestant pastors, holding my five-month old daughter on my lap and discussing the issue of abortion. This couldn't be me. Why was I doing this? What was my motivation?

I visited a Presbyterian church, which was close to my house. The pastor was very nice, listened attentively, but excused himself from any commitment for even a small meeting with his congregation. I visited a large Baptist church and spoke to one of its pastors. I was received cordially. We had a brief discussion about handicapped children, and then our request to speak there was turned down, also. I subsequently visited a Lutheran church. They agreed to a meeting, which went very well, as I remember.

Since my church already had one of the founders of the Right to Life League actively working there, I called another Catholic pastor. Here is where I was greeted with what was to become the "standard" reactions to our requests for meetings or sermons, or for even just distributing information to church members. I was told, in no uncertain terms, that this subject was much too controversial, and that this pastor wasn't interested in disturbing his flock. At least, he was up-front with us. What we were greeted with, subsequently, in Catholic churches, were pastors who were glad to support us in private, were glad to encourage us to be activists behind the scenes, but who were always cautious of anything too public. They were afraid that anything perceived as coming from them directly might cause trouble, might offend someone.

Later on, in answer to an appeal from lay Catholics for leadership in the pro-life movement, Cardinal Joseph Bernardin of Chicago, initiated the "seamless garment" approach. He said in a speech that abortion alone should not frame the right to life issue, but the rights of humans of all ages and circumstances should be highlighted. This should include laws against euthanasia, the threat of nuclear warfare, compassion for the handicapped and the elderly, etc. The Cardinal wouldn't have to get out of his comfort zone about the abortion issue, and neither would his bishops and priests. His remarks would appear to be non-judgmental and enlightened (i. e., uncontroversial, compassionate, modern) while he still supported his church's teaching that all life is precious. The effect was permission for all Catholic clergy to remain sheltered and to avoid, directly, the most basic issue of protecting life from its very beginning, from conception.

Of course, I don't disagree with the right to life for all human beings. I just disagree with the purpose and end result of his statements. If all Catholics had been hearing from about 1970 on, from their cardinals, bishops, and priests that the most basic right to life for the unborn was in jeopardy, and that we needed to pray and take action, we would see a much different attitude about abortion today. By watering down the debate so that the clergy could be protected from addressing the "sin" of abortion from the pulpit, the momentum and the leadership was lost, and the opportunity was lost to impact the entire country, as well.

Mainline pro-life activism has emanated from, and continues to be generated by, laymen, (especially Catholic women) who have been joined now by people of all faiths. Although abortion is not only a religious issue, the fact that God-centered people are the ones to take an active role in the fight for human rights is not surprising. Currently, pastoral leadership is still missing, and I have problems with statements like the following from a priest, whom I basically agree with on most other women's issues, Monsignor Paul Hayes: He said in his book, *The Gifts and Power of Woman*,[4] that it is up to Catholic women to take the lead in these matters. I don't think Catholic women should be alone in this endeavor, as they have been, without leadership from their pastors. For twenty-three years women have led the way in the pro-life movement. Many of their men have stood beside them, either actively taking part or being at-home support. However, our priests, bishops, and cardinals (not all, of course) have stood in the shadows, saying, in effect, "You go out there and tell them about abortion and the harmful effects of this sin. We will stand back, and let you speak. We don't want to become controversial."

I attended a meeting a few years ago for representatives of Respect Life Groups , (lay people who act as liaisons between the Catholic Archdiocesan office and their particular parishes on life issues) where the priest who heads this office in Los Angeles, was answering questions from the assembly. I asked why we haven't received more leadership from the pulpit, why there aren't more involved and active pastors, especially. Monsignor answered with surprising candor (I think he also surprised himself). He said that pastors needed to be *popular*, they needed not to offend or alienate their congregations. A general, concerted gasp was heard throughout the assembly. Popular? Popular? Since when is it the role of the parish priest or pastor to be popular? I always thought he was there to lead his congregation toward holiness. Where is he when we need him? In the shadows? Great!

Some of us had known or suspected this, and were surprised to hear the truth admitted publicly and others, new to pro-life action, were shocked. When Monsignor heard this gasp, he tried to further explain that pro-life activism should come from the laity. We, in turn, tried to explain that we needed leaders among the clergy. We felt that there would be much more enthusiasm and interest in the Catholic community for pro-life information and action if our priests would only speak out on Sundays and at other times. To ask for sermons and guidance from our priests did not seem like much to ask. I'm sorry to say that he either didn't understand our point or he chose to remain in his comfort zone.

I experienced similar feelings of incredulity and dismay when I was seated in a meeting with religion teachers in a respected Catholic girls' school, where we were discussing our (Pregnancy Center's) request to have our speakers come to their religion classes. After all, Planned Parenthood, had spoken to their students!  The following reaction was voiced by the Department Director of Religion, "But, we might offend some of these young women if we speak about abortion. Some of them have had abortions, and even some of their mothers have had abortions. Not all of our students are Catholic!"

I almost jumped out of my chair on that one. First of all, why would I send my child to a Catholic school and not expect her to learn Catholic doctrine? If non-Catholic parents want their daughters to get the excellent academic education offered by this institution, then I'm sure they can't complain about the religious education included.

And to say that it might hurt the girls' feelings if their mothers or they had had abortions is a spurious argument. Women who have had abortions want to talk about the experience. They want to get it out in the open. They want healing of their grief and their guilt. To continue the fantasy that it wasn't a mistake, that it wasn't hurtful, that a death didn't occur, only continues and reinforces their pain. And, if they truly feel no regret, grief or guilt, then how will it hurt them?

Pro-abortion activists accuse the Church of mind control in this area, when really we don't often hear about the most important issue of our time in our churches. We only hear about it from dedicated Catholics who continue educating and keeping alive the teachings against abortion, in spite of their priests, rather than alongside them. This situation saddens and bewilders me.

Anne Roche Muggeridge, a Canadian Catholic, had this to say, in her book, *The Desolate City: Revolution in the Catholic Church:*[5]

> *"Lay people have until recently, for instance, been the whole strength of the anti-abortion movement. Faithful to the mystery of the Incarnation and the divine human continuity, unflagging in the face of hostility, and even open opposition from the Catholic Theological and Social Justice offices. Except for self-serving politicians, Brian*

*Mulroney, John Turner, and Ed Broadbent in Canada, Geraldine Ferraro, Mario Cuomo, and Edward Kennedy in the United States, the lay Catholic, no matter how liberal in every other way, tends to remain adamant on this issue. What is more, the anti-abortion crusades has layed a solid base of ecumenical cooperation among Orthodox Christians, and has kept one bridge open on which bishops and others can escape back to the Catholic cosmology."*[6]

I was surprised to learn recently that 35% of the population in Los Angeles is Catholic. According to the Catholic Directory, the census for the year 1992[7], there are in the Los Angeles Diocese alone 3,527,481 Catholics. Whether that figure represents "practicing" Catholics, (those who attend Mass and receive the sacraments regularly) only, or those who traditionally are from a Catholic family but do not actively participate, is never quite clear in these kinds of polls. However, the point is that the Christian Church, Catholic or Protestant, could be the very real influence it is accused of being, if it only would.

As an example, in November of 1992, in California we were asked to vote on the issue of assisted suicide by medical personnel, Proposition 161. It was narrowly defeated. I believe that it was defeated only because a very real, organized effort was put forth by the leadership of the Catholic Church to educate its members about the true nature of this insidious "convenient death" plan.

Could it be that the concerted effort to defeat this assisted suicide bill was made because priests understood that they might be very ill someday, and they might not want someone else deciding when they should be assisted in dying? Could it be that because they will never have to face, personally, an unwanted pregnancy, they aren't as concerned?

The clergy, seemingly, do not understand that women who have had abortions need to face the sin and their grief and, thereby, begin the healing process. Rather than making their church members uncomfortable by discussing and preaching against abortion, priests could lead them, give them guidance, and, thereby, be true teachers and healers. To say that priests have to be non-controversial and well-liked prompts me to serious prayer for the souls of our "popular""clergy.

I truly believe that if the three and a half million Catholics in Los Angeles would hear only five or six sermons per year about the sanctity of human life, this city would have a more active pro-life outlook about abortion.

How about this at Sunday masses? "My dear brothers and sisters in Christ, the act of abortion takes the life of an unborn, innocent child, who is made in God's image. What a grievous sin this is! God is a loving and forgiving Father, but he is also a just God. If you or a loved one has been involved in an abortion, seek God's forgiveness. And actively work to educate this country about the abortion lie."

Christ asked us to love God and our neighbor. What better way to love than to help someone who has a crisis pregnancy? What better way to love than to help someone who has had an abortion face the grief and the guilt that eventually comes? What better way to help her deal with spiritual and emotional suffering--name the sin, and then help her to heal?

Or this? "I say to you, my brothers and sisters in Christ, that your disregard for human life in its mother's womb is scandalous! You must get back on the track of decency and responsible behavior. You must consider how precious is each human life. How can you condone and actively fight for a *right* to kill?" It's true that human circumstances are very often difficult, and sometimes seem impossible, but circumstances can be changed. Behavior can be changed. A woman who gets pregnant and has an abortion, usually has a second or a third one, too. Why? Because there haven't been any major changes in her behavior, and she is able to validate the first abortion by the second or the third. And so, the deadly behavior continues.

Just as there are comfortable priests and nuns, there are,

also, heroes and heroines among their ranks. The outspoken pro-life Catholic clergy are superheroes in my book. They are not popular with their moderate, keep-a-low-profile brothers and sisters in the clergy, and, of course, they are maligned by the pro-abortion press and their own moderate congregations. Some of the most well-known are Cardinal John O'Connor of New York, who goes against some very mighty press and has suffered the indignities of blasphemous behavior in his beautiful St. Patrick's Cathedral by Act-Up activists. Father Paul Marx heads an international organization, dealing with abortion and life issues. Bishop Austin Vaughn has publicly stood against abortion many times. Pope John Paul II, of course, has been eloquently outspoken about the sanctity of life. And, Mother Teresa of Calcutta has said: "My special prayer is that we will have a deep love for this gift of God, the child. For the child *is* the greatest gift of God to the world...and to each one of us."

Less well known, but heroes nonetheless are my favorite local priests and one sister. Father Peter Irving, who has been arrested and jailed for standing in front of the doors of an abortion clinic is a humble, courageous man. Father Thomas Cusack, a Columban father, speaks out, encourages us, and prays daily against abortion. Father Alex Chung came to our church as a new priest, and had the courage to speak out about the sin of abortion. He also actively supported pro-life education and prayer against abortion for our congregation. Sister Marcella is a beautiful, giving woman who was imprisoned for her sin of standing in front of an abortion clinic. The late Bishop Carl Fisher of the Los Angeles Archdiocese was an eloquently outspoken pro-life priest, one of the few black bishops in our country. He knew that minorities and low-income families are especially targeted by the pro-abortion activists.

We now have Christians from many different churches standing with their Catholic brothers and sisters. Here, too, the pro-life leadership has come mainly from the laity. They have some wonderfully outspoken pastors, however. Locally, in the

Los Angeles area, we have Reverend Tom Cizmar, a Lutheran. He has placed his pastoral career on the line by standing up for life in front of abortion clinics. Pastor Bob Ver Burg, a quiet and caring man is on the Board of the Right to Life League, where he encourages and inspires us. Here in the San Fernando Valley, Jack Hayford of Church on the Way has been eloquent on the pro-life issue.

Incidentally, the press characterizes all of these fine people as *right-wing fundamentalists*, and uses the term as an all-encompassing pejorative for people who believe in the Ten Commandments and read the Bible. Nothing could be farther from the truth, but it serves the press well to do so. They paint anyone who has a moral or religious world-view with the broad brush of radicalism, portraying them as members of a conspiracy to take over the government. The truth is that Christians who speak out against abortion do so from their deepest convictions, not because they want to overthrow any government.

Just as I talked about the comfort zone that clergy find for themselves, there is also the comfort zone for practicing Catholic, Protestant, and Jewish laymen who don't want to ask or know the truth about abortion. If they did, then they might have to do something about it, but if they say I'm personally opposed, but I don't think the government should make laws against abortion, then they can feel they've done their part.

The irony of the situation is that if the Church were as truly involved or "pro-active" as the media and pro-abortion activists try to portray there might be a little more unity and a lot more influence on people's minds and hearts. The Church does us no favors when it looks the other way. But, if the Church continues to remain silent, while its individual members try to carry on without leadership and only "behind-the-scenes" support, my grandchildren may never hear how a moral society should treat all of its members or that a stable, loving family is the cornerstone of our nation.

In "The Church Search," by Richard N. Ostling, an article which appeared in *Time Magazine*, April 5, 1993, the author quotes a Methodist minister, D. Stephen Long, of Divinity School at Duke University, who commented that he rejects the notion that ministers need to keep people happy and the "pews filled."

> " 'A pastor has to shake things up,' he says. 'The point isn't to accommodate self-centeredness but to attack it. If you don't, then the Gospel becomes just one more commodity we seek to package.' "[8]

What about our Jewish brothers and sisters? Where do they stand in all of this? It seems that only the observant, Orthodox Jew considers the sanctity of life to apply from conception to natural death. Rabbi Daniel Lapin is founding Rabbi of the Pacific Jewish Center in Venice, California, and president of Toward Tradition, whose activities he directs from Mercer Island, Washington. He says what needs to be said for Christian and Jew alike:

> *"Religious and observant Jews, on the other hand, constitute a fountain-head of conservative principles. Ronald Reagan won an overwhelming proportion of the orthodox Jewish vote. Unlike liberals, these Jews know that what threatens their survival is not Christianity but an American population with no religion at all. They must now open dialogues and form alliances with religious Christians. When all Jews recognize the benefits of our authentic heritage and finally realize that Judaism and certain kinds of liberalism are incompatible, we will start doing more good for America. We shall then once again be the kind of Jews President John Adams spoke of when he labeled us 'a most Essential element for civilizing the nations.' "*[9]

Rabbi Lapin stated it so well. Now, if only Jews and Christians alike heard this from all of their pastors, we would see some positive changes--some positive leadership. I fear for those clergy who stand in the shadows, hoping to stand clear of controversy, hoping not to offend, continuing their popularity at all costs. I fear for them and the families they are supposed to guide.

---

[1] John Jefferson Davis, *Abortion & the Christian*, Presbyterian and Reformed Publishing Co., Phillipsburg, NJ, 1984, p. 77.
[2] Bernard Nathanson, M.D., *Aborting America*, Doubleday & Company, Inc., Garden City, New York, 1979, p. 52.
[3] Ibid, p. 174.
[4] Msgr. Paul J. Hayes, *The Gifts & Power of Woman*, Daughters of St. Paul, Boston, 1987, p. 79.
[5] Anne Roche Muggeridge, *The Desolate City: Revolution in the Catholic Church*, Harper & Row, 1986
[6] Ibid., pp 166 & 167.
[7] Religion Section, "Los Angeles Catholic Census," *Los Angeles Daily News*, May 8, 1993.
[8] Richard N. Ostling, quoting Stephen D. Long, in "The Church Search," *Time Magazine*, April 5, 1993, Time-Life Publishers, p. 48.
[9] Rabbi Daniel Lapin, "Why are so Many Jews Liberal?" in *Crisis Magazine, a Journal of Lay Catholic Opinion*, April, 1993, pp. 10,11.

## *Toward a New Feminism*

"This day I call heaven and earth as witnesses against you that I have set before you life and death, blessings and curses. Now choose life, so that you and your children may live and that you may love the Lord your God, listen to his voice, and hold fast to him. For the Lord is your life, and he will give you many years in the land he swore to give to your fathers, Abraham, Isaac and Jacob."

_____Deuteronomy 30:19.

I have had two recurring daydreams over the years. Sometimes I use them to escape and sometimes just because it's fun to wonder, "What if?"

In one of my dreams I am a successful career woman. This picture probably developed from the "glamorous" ad-agency job I had when I was in my early twenties. For three and a half years I worked on the thirteenth floor of the Prudential Building in Chicago. At that time, it was the tallest building around. Across Lake Shore Drive, an apartment building was being constructed on the beautiful lakefront. This high-rise building, with a glass-domed pool on the outside, which was very chic at that time, is where I see myself living in this particular dream. I picture my eighteenth floor apartment in subdued, evening light. The furniture is soft browns and beiges, and the kitchen is small and cute--just the place for me to cook gourmet meals and impress handsome, exciting men and interesting women friends. From my love seat I can look out over the northern shore of the lake and if I turn my head to the left I can see the lights of the city and the toy cars dotting their way south on the Drive.

I am a single, career woman with many friends, an interesting job, and a self-assurance about what I do, who I am, and what my goals are. I walk to work on even the coldest days, just because it's only a few blocks away on Michigan Avenue. It's almost perfect, of course. Daydreams can be that way. It's full of sparkling sunshine on the lake in the late Spring and twinkling, snowy Christmas lights during the holiday season.

I'm never quite at peace in my perfect picture, however. I always have the feeling that there is a puzzle-piece missing. I hope it's not a husband or children. I hope that if this scenario had become my reality I would have found the missing piece. Maybe this would be just a nice place to go for a vacation, I eventually decide.

In my other imagined place I am on the second floor of a large home in a bedroom with many windows. The room is painted white and yellow and the soft curtains are blowing in, reaching toward my high, four-poster bed. I am sitting at a white desk, writing. Next to me is a white rocking chair. I pause and I look out the window nearest to me. I see a beautiful, sloping green lawn, that ends at the banks of a blue stream. There are several tall elm trees, but none obscures my view of the sunlight or the laughing children playing on the lawn. I am both at peace and moved by my feelings of love for the children and of my love for God and his wonderful creations. I think I'm writing a letter or a "great book." I'm not sure that the children are mine, but I love them, though I always seem to worry a little about the fact that I have placed the children so far from me in this particular dream.

Neither of these fantasies is true, of course. The feelings I fleetingly experience about them are different each time. The realities of who I became, a wife, a mom, a crisis pregnancy and post-abortion counselor, are probably a lot more interesting than my dreams.

I think women can have the best of both worlds. But, we have been too long defined by a society that wanted us to be kept in *our place*. And, now, we are being defined by feminists who seek empowerment, rather than equality. Unfortunately, included in this feminist agenda, is a contempt for women who choose the traditional roles of wives and mothers.

I'd like us all to consider a new type of feminism, one that celebrates women, nourishes their qualities and abilities, and seeks equality. Along with this, I want us to honor Moms who choose to be Moms only. I think we need to begin with our sons and daughters, our mothers, our friends, ourselves.

We learn our traditional gender roles from our families, in the first place. And then we learn from the world around us as we mature, as we are influenced by individuals outside of our families. There is a great song that comes from the musical, *South Pacific*, that demonstrates how we learn some things. "You've Got to Be Taught," is about racial prejudice, and how the youngest of us is taught to hate and fear anyone who is different. But the lyrics could very well be used when speaking about how we learn our feminine or masculine roles. The message of the song is that we aren't born with certain prejudices, but we are taught.

We are taught that little Timmy doesn't play with dolls (give him some toy soldiers or guns) and little Jennifer doesn't defend her rights by arguing or fighting (she must learn to compromise and adjust). And then, as we get into our teens, boys are urged, especially in high school to compete in sports and to prepare for college. Girls are not always so motivated. Then, later on, when we begin our own families, men are encouraged to be the leaders, the careerists. Women still are seen as the natural housekeepers, cooks and nurturers.

I couldn't believe what I was hearing one day, many years ago, when I attended a Retreat Day for women. The priest, a Father Love (or Dove, I forget which), as he discussed the differences between men and women, said that men aren't cut out to clean toilets. My blood pressure certainly must have gone up several notches. "Not made to clean toilets?" "But women are predestined to do that?" my brain shouted. I wasn't brave enough at that time to verbalize my anger and disbelief. I left after the lunch break. I was not a feminist, but deep within me I knew that this was one of the silliest things I had ever heard. The sad part about it is that I think he really believed what he said.

Simone de Bouvier, said in her book, *The Second Sex*, the following:

> "To gain the supreme victory, it is necessary, for one thing, that by and through their natural differentiation men and women unequivocally affirm their brotherhood."[1]

How can women begin to affect this change? This depends, of course, where we are at the moment in our individual lives. Michael and I have been married for twenty-seven years, and have four children, three girls and a boy. I believe, subconsciously, we always raised our children with an example of sharing roles and chores. I think Michael was a feminist before I was. He always did as much as he could to share the burdens of parenthood. He was always willing to change diapers, hold a crying infant, or go to the store for some forgotten items. An infant needs to be held, talked to, hugged, fed and have his diapers changed by Dad. When they are older, daughters need interaction and leisure time with their fathers, just as the boys do.

When a young girl begins the transition into womanhood

she needs her father to affirm that she is attractive and that she's interesting to be around. A simple, "You look nice today, Susan," is all that is needed. Or, a small non-birthday gift given to tell her she's special and feminine is important. Or, if she is interested in basketball, or soccer, or U2 or The Beatles, a Dad who is involved even in the smallest way will see that she has interests that are important to him, also.

I remember how much I enjoyed a very unusual dinner with my Dad one time. My mother had to go out of town for a few days when I was about fifteen. I truly can't remember where my two younger brothers were. Maybe she took them along. But, I remember my father treated me to a rather nice dinner in a lovely restaurant. We talked, as if we were both adults--pleasant, non-serious, conversation. Just an enjoyable, grown-up time. In the interest of total honesty, I think I had tried to cook for Dad the night before, and it had been close to a disaster. But, whatever the reason was doesn't matter. I loved our dinner, anyway.

Once children are into their teens they need all the help and affirmation they can get. They need it at home, at school, at church, and wherever they spend their free time. They need it in the music, television, and movies they are surrounded by. They need it in the books they read, and the magazines, textbooks, and library books that are published with teens in mind.

Teen girls, as well as teen boys, are striving to find out who they are, where they fit in. They must find out how they fit into their social environment. Are they pretty enough, are they smart enough, are they popular enough? What a struggle! I would never go back to that time again. And I lived in an easier, less-pressured era.

Teen girls and boys need to pay attention to grooming, with an emphasis on attractiveness-- not how to be the sexiest, but how to be their best. Girls need to be taught, in an age-appropriate manner, both make-up application, if they need it, and how to choose clothes. Even the most outlandish, bizarre fashion or makeup fad can be a modified version that would allow a teen girl to be *with it*. (I have seen orange and black-striped hair, and fishnet blouses worn over black bras on young girls who attend the middle school across the street from my home. Where are their parents? How do teachers keep their minds on teaching? How do the kids keep their minds on learning?)

If young women are able to learn who they are during their teen years, without defining themselves by the number of young men they have bedded, they can then make decisions about their futures when the opportunities present themselves. Whether marriage or career becomes most important in their lives, each stable, self-confident young person can make good decisions.

Marriage is a good, affirming way of life if men and women recognize that women are equal in the partnership. A woman should not sign on to be the one and only dishwasher or housekeeper. There should be a 50-50 deal in child-raising and discipline, infant care and baby-sitting, financial planning, and bill-paying.

Marriage should not be stifling or enslaving. It should afford both men and women even more freedom than they had as a single adult, an expanding of their possibilities and talents. Even children can be mind-expanding and fulfilling, rather than just a sacrifice and financial burden. To carry within her body the child she will eventually nurture, educate, and love, and then to be able to see that child achieve independence, is a privilege, not a burden. And, for a man to join her equally (even when she's pregnant) in these experiences is necessary for emotionally healthy kids.

What about women who would like to do both--be a Mom and have an interesting career or vocation? Women can have it all, family and career. I don't believe that both can be engaged in fully *simultaneously*, however. And, an abortion will not save a career.

Frederica Mathewes-Green said in an article, "Abortion and Women's Rights:"

*"Women's rights are not in conflict with their own children's rights; the appearance of such a conflict is a sign that something is wrong with our society. When women have the sexual respect and employment flexibility they need, they will no longer seek the substitute of the bloody injustice of abortion."*[2]

Attitudes and actual workplace conditions and flexibility must change, however. What is valuable needs to be defined. Is the only reason a woman returns to work for economic reasons? Or is she returning to work to nurture herself, to develop and contribute her talents? Mrs. Green continues in her article,

*"...Both parents can also benefit from more flexibility in the work place: allowing parents of school-age children to set their hours to coincide with the school day, for example, or enabling more workers to escape the expenses of office, commute, and child care by working from home. We must also welcome women back into the work force when they want to return, accounting for their years at home as valuable training in management, education, and negotiation skills."*[3]

Moms who wait until their children are at least 3- or 4-years old, and who are willing to look for the job or career that will allow them to work part-time or in the home, can have it all, eventually. After all, the average woman's life span is fairly long. Going back to work after age 35 still gives a woman many productive years for a career. A woman who chooses to work first, and then later on has a family and stays at home, should also be supported.

Not every woman, however, is suited for child raising or even childbearing. And that woman should be no less valued for her contribution to our multi-dimensional society. A career woman who chooses that deliberately over marriage and family needs good, nurturing friends and a society that praises and supports her, in whatever her chosen field.

I would like to see all young girls mature into adults who like themselves; women who won't necessarily seek empowerment over men, but rather equal opportunity and recognition. The new feminist would celebrate the differences between men and women, but would experience the personal and societal support to be successful in a career and marriage, and find fulfillment in both, or in just one of those roles.

I believe, wholeheartedly, that it is a woman's right to pursue a career. But, if she has a husband and children, they need to be included in decisions affecting the family. The anger and frustration of women, up to now, have been rooted in the fact that husbands have not included wife and family in the equation when their business decisions needed to be made. This lack of consideration is what needs to be changed. The kingship needs to become a limited democracy, where a wife's goals and choices are equally examined and considered. Although I don't advocate children having a clear vote, certainly utmost care and consideration for the welfare of children must be a priority. Some feminists will rail against these insipid, conciliatory ideas. Some plainly want empowerment, period.

In *Backlash:The Undeclared War Against American Women*, Susan Faludi, is clearly angry because she sees a loss of motivation, a compromise in the feminist quarter:

> *"As the backlash has gained power, instead of fighting and exposing its force, many women's groups and individual women have become part of the fitting into its fabricated backdrop. Feminist-minded institutions founded a decade earlier, from The First Women's Bank to Options for Women, camouflaged their intent with new, neutral-sounding names; women in colleges have claimed they are only interested in "family issues," not women's rights; and career women with ivy-league degrees have eschewed the feminist label for public consumption. Instead of assailing injustice many women have learned to adjust to it. Instead of getting angry, they have become depressed. Instead of uniting their prodigious numbers, they have splintered and turned their pain and frustration inward, some in starkly physical ways."*[4]

I think Faludi seeks nothing less than a matriarchy--no compromises, no fraternizing with the enemy.

A couple of friends, who knew I was writing a book about women told me I must review two movies: *Thelma and Louise*, and *Shirley Valentine*. I, dutifully, rented the videotapes. Both movies were interesting contrasts, and somewhere in the middle might be found a true feminist outlook.

Thelma and Louise hated men, destroyed them in their hell-bent path, and eventually destroyed themselves. They took on male attributes with a gun in hand and proceeded to vent their anger and frustration on the *enemy*.

Shirley Valentine had a dullard for a husband, who thought she existed to cook his meals on time and to his specifications. In a nasty scene, which changed Shirley's outlook on her empty marriage, hubbie dumped a meal that he is not pleased with in her lap. She runs away from her boorish husband and her dreary apartment in London, to Greece, where she meets the resident gigolo, has an affair, and decides to stay. She takes a job as a cook at the seaside resort that was the scene of her brief love affair. Her husband, after many phone calls begging her to come back, eventually joins her there. The last scene is Shirley Valentine, sitting with her husband, watching a very romantic sunset.

Shirley may or may not have solved her problem. We're not quite sure. The end of the movie offers hope, possibly, as she and hubbie sit quietly watching the Greek sunset, but I was never sure she really understood the change she was capable of making. Does he get out of his dullard role, does he come to the realization that she is not his property? Or do they go on as before, only in Greece this time? Remember, she is still cooking.

I'd like to propose that real freedom and equality for women lies in common sense, determination, some compromise, and a realistic outlook on what can and can't be changed. Women do have choices--they need only to act on them. Marriage, career, children, or all of the above? How to decide?

Some women have felt society's pressure to be mothers, even though they weren't really ready to have children. The result is frustration and anger. In a book, *Mother's Day is Over*,[i] by Shirley L. Radl, the author details her mistaken motherhood. It was a very honest book. Truly, she should not have had children. Ideally, she should have been living in a society that accepted her non-maternal instincts and accepted and valued her for who she is and what was the more natural career for her.

*"...We tend to overlook the fact that we are not all equally suited for parenthood, anymore than we are for teaching school or playing various sports. Matters of temperament, age, health and competing interests, to mention just a few, are considerations in determining whether or not to have children."*[ii]

Today, however, a reverse situation seems to be the politically-correct mentality. Mothers who choose to be mothers only are not respected, as in: "Do you work?" "No, I stay at home with my kids." Not work? Not work hard? Mothering is very demanding work, indeed.

E. James Lieberman, a psychiatrist, was quoted in *Report of the Commission on Population Growth and the American Future*:[iii]

*"The plain truth is that being a mother is the most important, difficult and demanding of careers. At stake is the very life of another*

*human being--and almost total responsibility for that life during its formative years. E. James Lieberman, a psychiatrist, formerly with the National Institute of Mental Health writes: 'Child-rearing is the most difficult task that most ordinary mortals will ever undertake. It is the first priority of this and every nation; costly to do well and costlier to neglect.' We are not doing a good enough job, but the challenge is sobering."*[iv]

Wives and mothers who are companions, nurturers, counselors, teachers, secretaries and cooks are truly worthy of praise and recognition. Unfortunately, the choice of staying at home with one's children has been disdained, sometimes causing those who would pursue it with joy and contentment, to look at their more fashionable sisters with envy and feelings of inferiority. Why can't we accept both lifestyles, both careers? Both are valuable. Both should be applauded.

If a woman pursues her career first, and then has children, she needs to be home with them during the early years (or her husband needs to be). It doesn't mean that she stops using her gifted mind, or that her brain shuts down. She can develop other talents and interests. With the easy access of home computers, she can still pursue her chosen field, part-time, though she may have to wait a few years to climb a corporate ladder. If her career, and not just the big salary, truly interests her, a few years at home will not be a disadvantage.

Our brains are wonderful things: if we keep them exercised and interested they serve us well. My own personal suggestion for the mothering years is "Get rid of your television set!" It's an annoyance, an intrusion, a poor teacher, a poor baby sitter, and just not necessary. It's a waste of time, and with today's fare your children and you and your husband are better off without it. Do I have a television set in my home?. Yes, I've had to compromise, but I rarely watch it. I have more interesting and fulfilling things to do.

Full-time career and full-time Mom? Some can do it, as

said. Good Luck to them. But, I would like to promote the "two-separate careers" plan. If we marry at age 22 or 23, even if we have three children in ten years' time, at age 37, for example, we can go, full-time, into a previously chosen or new career. Valuable years haven't been lost. We've just added dimension and breadth to our understanding, skills, and talents. If you wanted to be a billionaire, you might be at a disadvantage, but less-than-billionaire status doesn't mean you are a failure. If you have your health at this point, you can predictably look at 25 years or more of pursuing your career, of loving what you do.

Let's look at another situation. A woman marries, but she does not have children right away. She and her husband both have careers. She works until she's 34, and then gets pregnant. Great! She's got ten years in her chosen field, lots of experience, but now she's ready to try this new motherhood thing. Again, she has three children, and then at age 45 decides to return to work. She could easily have fifteen or twenty more years of career, and she's already had ten.

The error is made when women are unhappy because they aren't economic contributors to their marriage. Times are tougher, financially, for the family where only the husband is working. But the benefits to the marriage and family, in the long run, are immeasurable.

Rather than day care, what is needed is a tax break for women who work only in their homes. If a husband earns $40,000 a year for a family of five, at least $7200 per year should be deducted from his total income for his wife's domestic services. Let's look at those services realistically: child caretaker, cleaner, cook, chauffeur, shopper, secretary, bookkeeper, and so on. If that isn't worth three times $7200, I don't know what is. This deduction would allow each family to keep more of its actual earnings, and spend more of it. That can only be a plus for our nation's economy, besides.

Neither of these life plans is unrealistic or unworkable. I'm not into sacrifice as you may have noticed. I suggest that during our mothering years we continue to pursue our interests. The completely-involved mom who does little league, dance lessons, school volunteerism, gymnastics, etc. for her kids and denies herself her own time, her own pursuits and talents, is to be applauded. But, I sometimes wonder if she isn't subconsciously resentful and if her children and their accomplishments are "everything" to her. Will she be lost when they start leaving for college, careers, and marriage?

Most of us can do both, just not at the same time, and women should have the freedom to do just that. June Sochen talks about Eleanor Roosevelt's advice in her book, *Movers and Shakers*:

*"Considering women as persons must begin with women themselves, she reminded her readers. Always encouraging women to fulfill their human potential, she answered those who asked her whether wives should work by saying that they were asking the wrong question. The question should be: 'Are you able to carry on two full-time jobs? If you are healthy, well organized, and have a supportive husband, you will probably succeed.' If any of these factors are missing, Mrs. Roosevelt counseled, you will have problems."*[9]

There are only a few of us who are lucky enough to have all of those criteria in place, simultaneously, and then even fewer of us who are extraordinary enough to take advantage of it.

Simone de Beauvoir, in her book, [10]*The Second Sex*, talks about man as the "absolute," and woman as the "other."

De Beauvoir believes the idea of the "absolute" (man) and the "other" (woman) is detestable. She, indeed, bases her case for feminism on the dissolution of that difference. I agree, in part, but not with the idea of superiority or empowerment that she advocates. In her conclusion, however, is, possibly, the societal answer for the change that is needed.

*"If the little girl were brought up from the first with the same demands and rewards, the same severity, the same freedom, as her brothers, taking part in the same studies, the same games, promised the same future, surrounded with women and men who seem to her undoubted equals, the meanings of the castration complex and the oedipus complex would be profoundly modified. Assuming on the same basis of the father, the material and moral responsibility of the couple, the mother would enjoy the same lasting prestige; the child would perceive around her an androgynous world and not a masculine world. Were she emotionally more attracted to her father--which is not even sure -- her love for him would be tinged with a will to emulation and not a feeling of powerlessness; she would not be oriented for passivity,*

*authorized to test her powers in work and sports, competing actively with the boys. She would not find the absence of the penis--compensated by the promise of a child--enough to give rise to an inferiority complex; correlatively, the boy would not have a superiority complex if it were not instilled into him, and if he looked up to women with as much respect as to men. The little girl would not seek sterile compensation and narcissism and dreaming, she would not take her fate for granted; she would be interested in what she was doing, she would throw herself without reserve into undertakings."*[11]

Why can't the world consist of two "others" or two "ones?" Why can't women and men be equals? I think they can be. But both men and women need to change their perspectives.

Annette Baxter, in her book, *To Be A Woman in America*,[12] gives a positive example of paternal influence, in Jane Addams' relationship with her father:

*"...But the most crucial of her relationships with men may have been a woman's with her father. Jane Addams, founder of the Settlement House and lifelong champion of the underprivileged, attributed a shaping influence to her father's abhorrence of inequality and his rigorous honesty with himself."*[13]

Baxter notes another less positive aspect of patriarchal influence:

*"Yet fathers could be a source of irritation as well as inspiration, In "Woman's True Duty," an admonitory tale, which appeared in Miss Leslie's Magazine, the dutiful heroine asks of her moral counselor what she might do to her please her father, and is told: 'your father is fond of music. A song from you would delight him when he returns wearied from his counting-house. Yet, I have heard you refuse to sing for him.' The daughter's reply is couched in the polite accents of her time, but expresses a thoroughly contemporary impatience. 'That was wrong, I confess--but he always asks for old songs, such as were the fashion 30 years ago; if he would listen to my new music.'"*[14]

Indeed, if fathers only listened to new music, whatever it might be, by encouraging and actively participating in their daughters' education, sports activities, artistic pursuits, or music, young women would mature with a different view of themselves, their sexuality, their worth, and their ability to thrive in a chosen career or marriage relationship.

There would be fewer teen girls who think they must have sex because the boy has taken them out for a hamburger and a movie. Fewer women would be promiscuous because they wouldn't need to seek, in many men, the bonding, understanding, love, and friendship they did not receive from their fathers. There would eventually be a lot fewer women who long endure their abusive husbands or boyfriends.

Why should the more strident, power-seeking, revengeful feminism be reconsidered or revised? The most compelling reason is that it just isn't working. Feminists, today, seem to promote aggressiveness, anger, and resentment. It's an "us against them" type of mentality. Thelma and Louise are predominant. Sexual liberation and the freedom that was supposed to come from legal abortion has not materialized. Quite the opposite has occurred. Another form of repression has arisen, and women have bought into it. The irony is that men once again are the winners and women the losers.

Women told women they should be sexually free. Get involved with as many men as you like. Why choose marriage? Why not pursue (and bed) all the men who catch your eye? I ask, is this real freedom and equality? Their men feel no need to protect or love them, and no responsibility toward the children they might father with them. They never had a commitment or, heaven-forbid, a marriage license. When women agreed to "live together" first, without a wedding, they lost their freedom, not gained it!

Women need to understand that a free sexual lifestyle and abortion are *not* changing women's lives or society for the better. They need to consider that they have done nothing for women's advancement.

Surprisingly, I find myself standing with Betty Friedan, the founder of N.O.W., (National Organization of Women) on some issues, even though her pro-abortion stand is abhorrent. In her famous book, *The Feminine Mystique*,[15] she concluded:

# Toward a New Feminism

> *"...And when women do not need to live through their husbands and children, men will not fear the love and strength of women, nor need another's weakness to prove their own masculinity. They can finally see each other as they are. And this may be the next step in human evolution.*
>
> *"Who knows of the possibilities of love when men and women share not only children, home, and garden, not only the fulfillment of their biological roles, but the responsibilities and passions of the work that creates the human future and the full human knowledge of who they are? It has barely begun, the search of women for themselves. But the time is at hand when the voices of the feminine mystique can no longer drown out the inner voice that is driving women on to become complete."*[16]

Unfortunately, Friedan has been a leader in the pro-abortion movement. She wrote an introduction to the twentieth anniversary of her book. In an incongruous discussion of abortion and the need for it, she talked personally about her family:

> *"My daughter-in-law, Helen, is technically, at the moment, mostly a housewife. The baby was not exactly planned. There were difficult choices to be made, since both she and Jonathan, my younger son, had just finished college, after having dropped out for some years. One day last summer, when they'd brought the baby out to my house in Sag Harbor, Helen overheard me on the Supreme Court decision asserting women's rights to legal medical abortion. 'The right to abortion is very important to me,' said this post-feminist mother, nursing her baby. 'It's important knowing that we had the baby because we chose to.'"*[17]

On the very same page, Betty bubbles brightly and "profoundly:"

> *"And I, as a grandmother at last, am the envy of my friends, whose doctor/lawyer/banker daughters are too caught up in their careers to yet carry on the gene pool. With my beautiful, incredible grandbaby--such a beaming, bright bundle of energy, smiling at me with his father's big ears and dimples and his own blue eyes, so familiar, so intensely alive, so awesome a miracle--I*

*exult in the generation of life, though I have been too busy this year to baby-sit much.*"[18]

In other words, a baby is a baby if you want it, have room for it in your life, and aren't too much discomfited by his or her poor timing. Her daughter-in-law says that the most important thing is that they had the baby *because they chose to.*

Not! Wrong! The most precious thing is human life, her baby's *and* everyone else's. How very selfish of Helen to think that she need not be concerned for one-and-a-half million other pre-born babies who die every year because they are inconvenient! How sanctimonious of Betty to wax grandmotherly in the face of her friends' daughters who are *only* bankers and lawyers.

Who are these women with their double standards? All women should have equal rights, born and unborn. All are persons--all are precious. That a pre-born human being should have the right to life and be granted personhood on the whim of his mother is about as subjective and biased as one can possibly get! Where are the equal rights for the pre-born child?

If I could only convince Betty Friedan that the right to life for unborn children is so much more important, and must supersede, all of the women's equality issues. If I could only convince her that legal abortion has succeeded only in enslaving women further and annihilated whole generations of children in a frenzy of selfishness and infanticide. If only she would acknowledge that the abortion mentality has seriously damaged women, families, and our country. If I could only do all that, she and I could do great things together.

I propose that young girls be nurtured as human beings with potential for all things, motherhood included, if that path is chosen-- so that they can say, as adults: "I am a woman, I am part of mankind, I am equal with men, and I have certain inalienable rights. I can live without a man because I have grown up as an independent, valuable person, but I am open to a man as my husband and life partner, if I choose, if I find the right person. I know that I am not defined by my children or my husband, or the lack of either. I will accept and adapt, when and where I need to. But, I will always claim my rights, without harm to another. I am a woman and I can be all that I strive to be."

If we don't change things, especially changing our minds about our "rights" to abortion, the violence that continues to escalate in all areas of our society will eventually destroy this country. The abortion connection to this general violence is very real. When Roe v. Wade declared open season on our unborn citizens, giving women a right to kill their children because of a perceived *penumbra emanating from a right of privacy*, all of us became members of an endangered species.

God is the author of life--not physicians, judges, lawyers, clerics, teachers or legislators. We cooperate with God's plan when we conceive and become mothers and fathers. The gift of a human life is a wondrous thing, not a curse.

There are those who say we must change people's hearts and minds about the issue of abortion. That's true, but usually what is meant is that they want to wash their hands of the whole issue, so that they don't have to speak out. They say that there will always be abortion, that the government can't stop it, so we shouldn't even try to make abortion illegal again. And, I say that the Supreme Court made a serious error in 1973, and that if we don't turn back and correct our course where it made a wrong turn, we won't be able to change hearts and minds. As long as abortion is legal, it will be perceived as a moral option, a moral good.

When I ask women what they would do if abortion were *illegal*, they are always able to come up with an alternate plan. It is most often a life-giving, life-affirming plan that embodies hope for them and for their unborn children.

Feminists must continue to seek equal rights and respect for women, but they must include all of humanity in their quest, including their preborn sons and daughters. Loving and protecting the most innocent and vulnerable of us and then teaching our children that they are valued human beings is the beginning of true equality for all.

God is the giver of life, and that knowledge needs to be the foundation of a new feminism, a new path. So, choose life, as we are all, men, women, and preborn children, part of the family of man.

---

[1] Simone De Bouvier, *The Second Sex*, Alfred A. Knopf, NY 1952, p. 732

[2] Frederica Mathewes-Green, "Abortion and

Women's Rights," *ALL About Issues* magazine, published by American Life League, Virginia, March-April, 1992, p. 13.
[3] Ibid.
[4] Susan Faludi, *Backlash: The Undeclared War Against American Women*, Crown Publishers, Inc., NY 1991, p. 57.
[5] Shirley L. Radl, *Mother's Day is Over*, Charterhouse 1, NY 1973.
[6] *Report of the Commission on Population Growth and the American Future*, New American Library, New Am Library NY 1972, p. 126.
[7] Ibid.
[8] E. James Lieberman, "Informed Consent for Parenthood; Abortion and the Unwanted Children," *Calif. Comm. on Therapeutic Abortion*, Springer, NY'71, p.18., *Report of the Commission on Population Growth and the American Future*, New American Library, New Am Library NY 1972, p. 126.
[9] Ibid., p. 155.
[10] Simone de Beauvoir, *The Second Sex*, Alfred A. Knopf, NY 1952.
[11] Ibid., p. 726.
[12] Annette K.Baxter, *To Be A Woman in America, 1850-1930*, Times Books, NY 1978.
[13] Ibid., p. 136.
[14] Ibid.
[15] Betty Friedan, *The Feminine Mystique*, 20th Anniversary edition, W. W. Norton & Co., NY, 1983, p. 348.
[16] Ibid., pp. 377 & 378.
[17] Ibid., pp. xii & xiii.
[18] Ibid., p. xiii.

# EPILOGUE

In September of 1995, our chapter of the Right to Life League of Southern California celebrated its twenty-fifth anniversary with a dinner and a speech by Joseph Scheidler of the Pro-Life Action League. Mr. Scheidler had been named as the most influential pro-life acivist in the country by Ms. Magazine in June, when they put out an entire issue on "enemies of abortion." It was a wonderful evening. Joe Scheidler inspired us all to continue our work with Moms and unborn babies.

As I listened to him talk about our involvement since 1970, I realized that I, too, had been part of the pro-life movement for twenty-five years. In the weeks following, I was a bit down because I felt that I, personally, needed to feel more unity, to be more in-touch, with all of the pro-life groups in this country. I know that there are over three thousand centers like ours in the United States, and that we are bedrock organizations for the pro-life movement. I wanted to embrace and encircle all of them. I hoped that we could dialogue, interact and be strong for one another. Earlier, in June, I had visited a center in the small town of Montrose, Colorado. Why couldn't I visit more centers? Be a Johnny Appleseed, planting the seeds of unity--letting each group know that their daily stand against the culture of death is being repeated over and over again in many large cities and small towns across our country.

At about this same time, I heard the Amtrak commercials for their All Aboard America fares. For only $278.00 I could travel to an unlimited number of cities within a 30-day period. My friend, Mary Stevens, and I had talked about doing this together a few years ago. But now, because of her cancer, she would not be able to travel. I told her about my idea of going it alone. She had always been such a good friend and support for all of our pro-life work. Once again, she encouraged me and said, "Go for it!"

I visited the Crisis Pregnancy Centers of Greater Phoenix, the National Headquarters of Operation Rescue, in Dallas, Texas, the Pro-Life Action League (Joe Scheidler's group) in Chicago, three other pregnancy centers in Chicago, the

National Committee for a Human Life Amendment, the Christian Coalition, and the U. S. Senate in Washington, D.C.

I have not discussed Operation Rescue in this book, but I know many of the good people in O.R. At their headquarters in Dallas, I did not meet Norma McCorvey, Miss Roe. She was taking care of a sick friend the day I showed up at their office. But I did talk with Kirsten Breedlove, who had been the Director of several abortion clinics. I'd like to tell you her very powerful story.

Kirsten graduated from Nursing School at the age of 18 in Sherman, Texas. She began working at a small hospital in Sherman and was dating a doctor there. She went to a charity fundraising dinner with him one evening, and there met an interesting doctor who was wearing a Rolex watch. She was impressed with him and his watch, and the fact that he was sitting at the table designated for those who had donated the most money to this particular cause. Lamar Robinson was his name. He told Kirsten that he did hysteroscopies. (A hysteroscopy is a late-term abortion technique. I tried to find out more about this procedure, but even the National Abortion Federation was not familiar with it. The doctor must use some kind of a scope to see the baby while aborting it.) He needed a nurse, and he made an appointment with her.

Kirsten was sickened the first time she observed the procedure, because with the hysteroscopy technique you see the baby during the whole abortion procedure, as it is being dismembered. Even though this was upsetting to her, Robinson's obvious wealth and status impressed Kirsten.

Eventually, she found in the Yellow Pages, a clinic named A to Z Women's Services. It was a run-down facility, but they didn't do the hysteroscopy procedure. She went to work for them right away. Here is Kirsten's story:

> "I wanted the Director's job and eventually got it. I would do a lot of PR work. I would go to the schools. I would tell the girls not to tell their mothers. I was very fake and good to them so they would come back.
>
> "I got into drugs very heavily--cocaine intravenously. And it began to inhibit my work. I ended up telling the clinic that my father had

# Epilogue

*died and I left. I had only been there 6 months. I was gone for a year. I had stopped using drugs. Out of the blue, A to Z called me back. I didn't really want to be the Director anymore. For one thing, my clinic was the only free-standing clinic in Dallas. We had all the pro-lifers in front of our clinic. It was a pain. I ended up going back only as the Nursing Director, but within three months I was the Director again.*

"*I was only twenty-one years old. I had no administrative experience, but I was good. We saw the most patients, though we went as far as 25 weeks. We were the cheapest. Our late-term abortions were $1025, where some clinics are as high as $1595. We used two-day laminaria insertion. There were a lot of mistakes. A lot of torn uteruses, a lot of perforations. I sent five women in the last six months home with perforated uteruses. One woman lost her uterus. Our doctor was getting very shaky and was getting very accident prone. At one point, I found myself delivering a breech stillborn by myself because the doctor wouldn't answer my beeps. I had to be on call seven days a week, all hours.*

"*The pro-lifers were out in front of my clinic every day. This guy, Mark, was out in front and I'd try to get him with my car. He'd show me some crosses, but I would try to break them. I was a Catholic school girl. I didn't like them. I would call 911 and they would say, "Is it Mark again?" I could ask the police to come at any time. They saw us as the respectable ones. I went on TV when I was still working at the clinic and told them how terrible the pro-lifers were. It was great PR, and it de-sensitized people to what was going on in the clinic.*

"*I started to have a friendship with Mark. I was using drugs again, but he gave me hope that there was a better way of life. I was the only one doing sonograms and I eventually would turn the screen toward the women and I would show them their babies. It became harder and harder to come to work.*

"*It must have been a God thing. Satan felt me getting closer to God. I ended up in the hospital with a drug overdose. I was very sick. This lady, Jill Bousha, started to call me. She was weird. She would tell me she loved me and would pray for me. She has three little daughters. The doctors told me that I would probably die of the staph infection on my arm where the needle tracks were. My arms were a mess. Operation Rescue sent me a bouquet of flowers with Jeremiah 11 on it. Five days later I checked out of the hospital.*

"*When I went back to the apartment, Jill came and prayed with me. This was on March 26, 1995. She and her husband let me come and live with them. We read the Bible, and I started walking women out of the clinic. I told them to talk to the pro-lifers. My boss found out I was doing this after the clinic went bankrupt. I would say, 'If you'll just go, I'll give you your sonogram money back.' It wasn't really clear to the owner that I was the reason for the bankruptcy, but I lost my job when they shut down.*

"*I was offered jobs at many other abortion clinics. I've been helping out at Jill's crisis pregnancy center. I still have dreams, and I battle with drugs daily. There aren't many exits. Satan controls me with drugs. I was going to AA meetings daily. I'm working in a nursing home--I'll start Monday. I still have dreams of the POC (products of conception) room. I've gotten so many people started in the abortion business.*

"*My Mom's not a Christian. She thinks I just found a new drug. I was a Catholic school girl, but my family really wasn't religious. I lived on the near North side of Chicago. I was abused as a child--sexually abused by my father. I'm slowly remembering things from my childhood. I have one sister who is in Sherman, married with kids, and my brother, who is a doctor in Lubbock. My family was not really close. I've learned about normal families from Jill and Mr. Bousha. I've learned that I don't have to fear him when he hugs me. I've only talked to my father once in the last four years. I've forgiven him and I told him that I did, but I don't need a relationship with him.*"

Kirsten, as I think she knows, has a long road to recovery ahead of her. She is currently attending AA meetings as a recovering drug addict, and trying to shape a career for herself using her nursing skills in a more positive way.

From Dallas, I traveled to Chicago. There I visited Joe Scheidler's Pro-Life Action League, the Women's Center on the West side of Chicago, Aid for Women in downtown Chicago, and the Loop Center, also in downtown Chicago. At each of these pro-life centers I was welcomed warmly and was able to determine, that even though we were all in different cities, different surroundings, with very different budgets, we all were essentially doing the same thing—saving Moms and babies from the terrible decision that would ruin both of their lives.

Then, after Thanksgiving, I went to Washington. While I was there I visited the National Committee for a Human Life Amendment (a Catholic bishops organization, dedicated to continuing the fight against abortion), and The Christian Coalition. (a national organization dedicated to making a Christian political difference) I was also lucky enough to

# Epilogue

witness speeches by Senators Orrin Hatch, Robert Smith, and Inhofe of Oklahoma in favor of HR 1833, the partial-birth abortion ban bill. Here is what happened in the Senate on December 5, 1995.

I arrived about three o'clock on Monday and took a seat in the Senate Gallery. This was my first time in the august chamber. It's very different than I had imagined because there are only one or two senators and their aides in the chamber at the time of the speeches. So, in fact, the senators are really speaking to the gallery and the C-Span television camera. The cameramen change shifts quite frequently because, as I observed, there is so little to do (the position of the camera is almost never changed) and the cameramen nod off sometimes. One would hope that none of them ever snores.

The abortion debate didn't begin until about 5:00 PM. It began with Senator Orrin Hatch's speech in favor of the ban. It was exciting for me to hear him in person. He has been a pro-life legislator from the State of Utah for many years. In fact, if we had been behind the "States' rights" bill that he introduced many years ago, we might be a lot farther along in the pro-life movement. I, and many other "purists," thought at that time that it was too much of a compromise. I now feel that we were wrong on that one. If states had been able to pass pro-life legislation for these many years, we would be much closer to changing hearts and minds.

Senator Robert Smith of New Hampshire, the senator who had introduced the partial-birth abortion (D and X) bill in the Senate, spoke next. He was eloquent in his impassioned argument for the ban. During the time he had the floor, he displayed the drawing of this revolting procedure. I was thrilled to hear him, and wished that I had been allowed to bring in my little tape recorder, but that is not allowed.

Barbara Boxer spoke next. She was quite dramatic in her argument to keep this late-term abortion procedure legal. She cited two examples of women who had testified in the Senate hearings. She used an enlarged photo of one of the women and her family. Barbara said that this woman might have died if she couldn't have availed herself of the D and X abortion. She repeated several times that this woman was a pro-life, Catholic Republican, as if that made everything all right.

Senator Inhofe from Oklahoma spoke next and refuted the two examples that Boxer had given. Neither woman cited had had the procedure that was in question. And, he said that there really are no life-threatening situations which would mandate that this procedure remain as a legal method of abortion.

The next day I decided to go back to the Senate office buildings and do a bit of lobbying. I visited about ten Senators, leaving them a note on our "Abortion Stops a Beating Heart," postcards. In Senator Kennedy's office I asked why he couldn't vote as his pro-life son had voted in the House of Representatives? In Jesse Helms office I just enjoyed the Southern hospitality and the Christmas tree that was already decorating the waiting area. In Senator Coverdell's (R-Georgia) office I spoke to his aide, who said he hadn't made up his mind yet. So, I gave him my Precious Feet pin (a universal pro-life symbol that is the exact size and shape of a ten-week pre-born's feet). I noted later that he had, indeed, voted for the ban.

This bill, known as HR 1833, eventually was passed by an overwhelming margin by the House of Representatives and the Senate. The President, however, vetoed this law on April 10, 1996. His "handlers" made sure that he was surrounded by women who had had a D and X, saying it was their only option.

In response to an article in the *Los Angeles Times*, "The Politics of Heartbreak," in the Life and Style section of the May 8, 1996 edition, Murphy Goodwin, a Los Angeles obstetrician-gynecologist, who specializes in high-risk cases, and several other physicians wrote a letter to the *Times,* saying that there are no situations where a D and X (partial-birth) abortion is medically necessary. The *Times* didn't print it. Here are some of the misrepresentations in the article, along with the facts.

1. "…in most cases it (the fetus) has died before reaching the birth canal." **Fact**: There is no form of anesthesia or sedation administered to the mother which causes the death of the fetus in utero.

# Epilogue

2. "The excess amniotic fluid collecting in her uterus could have caused a rupture..." **Fact**: The problem of excess amniotic fluid accumulation affects hundreds of women in the Los Angeles area alone at any one time. Rupture of the uterus is not a recognized complication of excess amniotic fluid.
3. "...and if the fetus died in utero, dangerous toxins could have been emitted." **Fact**: Yes, there are risks to the mother if the dead fetus is retained in utero for more than one month. Even so, these risks can [be] and are managed every day by high risk pregnancy specialists in cases such as the death of one twin when the surviving twin is too small to deliver safely.
4. "Nothing could be done to save the babies, and as their conditions worsened, the risks to the mothers' health and future fertility grew." **Fact**: "We are not aware of any increased risk of carrying through such a pregnancy after late pregnancy diagnosis (the "sixth month" in the cases in the story) in the absence of other specific pregnancy-related diseases. The management of such cases is technically and emotionally challenging but there are other safe options besides the procedure these patients underwent.

# UPDATE

Since I finished this book in February of 1994, many things have changed on the national scene. I would like to update my readers with a list that is current as of April 1, 1996:

In Chapter 4, I spoke about **Joycelyn Elders as our Surgeon General.** I am pleased to report that she was forced to resign after she publicly advocated teaching masturbation in sex education classes, including those students under the age of ten. At this time, there is no Surgeon General, as the only appointee proposed by the President, Henry Foster, was not confirmed.

Sadly, we are one step closer to **legalized euthanasia** with a decision in favor of assisted suicide, handed down on March 6, 1996 by the U. S. Ninth Circuit Court of Appeals. From the *Los Angeles Times* newspaper of March 7, 1996, we learned that Judge Stephen Reinhardt, (appointed by Jimmy Carter) as one of an 8 to 3 majority, cited Roe v. Wade as a basis for his ruling that:

*"There is a constitutionally protected liberty interest in determining the time and manner of one's own death."*[1]

Judge Stephen Reinhardt wrote in his majority opinion:

" *'A competent, terminally ill adult, having lived nearly the full measure of his life, has a strong liberty interest in choosing a dignified and humane death rather than being reduced at the end of his existence to a childlike state of helplessness, diapered, sedated, incompetent...' 'If broad general state policies can be used to deprive a terminally ill individual of the right to make that choice, it is hard to envision where the exercise of arbitrary and intrusive power by the state can be halted.' Reinhardt's analysis relies heavily on language drawn from U.S. Supreme Court abortion cases because the issues have 'compelling similarities,' he wrote."*[2]

The judges who agreed with this ruling were: James Browning, Procter Hug, Mary Schroeder, Betty Fletcher, Harry Pregerson, Charles Wiggins, and David Thompson.

# Update

The dissenting judges were: Robert Beezer, Ferdinand Fernandez, and Andrew Kleinfeld.

Judge Robert Beezer wrote in his dissent:

> *"If physician-assisted suicide is made a constitutional right, voluntary euthanasia for weaker patients, unable to self-terminate, will soon follow."*[3]

Incidentally, Judge Reinhardt is married to Ramona Ripston, who is the head of the ACLU (American Civil Liberties Union), a leading advocate for legal abortion. The right to abortion, and now legal, assisted suicide, has made us a nation of pragmatic, violent people. We have only to look around to see the increase in child abuse, gang violence and murder, guns in our schools and on our streets, rape, assault, child abuse, and a general disrespect for life. Human life is cheap.

In Chapter 5, I spoke about **Jan, the schizophrenic mother,** whom we helped and then, later, intervened in order to procure a safer environment for her daughter. Jan called us about six months ago. She said that she just wanted to thank us for helping her at the time she was pregnant. She said that her daughter had been adopted, and that the new parents were letting her be a part of their daughter's life. Jan was back on the medication that allows her to live a more normal existence. She wanted to thank us, too, for helping her daughter.

In Chapter 6, <u>Used Women and Abortion,</u> I spoke about the abortion industry and its abuse of women. Not detailed there at the time, but having since come to light, is the fact that **in China, aborted fetuses are used as health food**. Detailed in several publications is the fact that doctors use and sell the nutrient-rich little bodies of aborted babies for the purposes of cannibalism. One reporter was offered some of the "products of conception," and then wrote about this atrocity.

In Chapter 6, I also talked about **Leane, who had had several abortions**, and then conceived at age 41. I am happy to report that Leane and her husband have a healthy, handsome son.

Also, in Abortion & the Medically-Correct, research of the **link between abortion and breast cancer** had not been reported at the time of my writing. Since then, several studies have reported a definite link. From a pamphlet that cites thirteen studies, published by Hayes Publishing,[4] an explanation is given that cancer cells can develop when a woman aborts, abruptly reversing, in a transitional stage, the new cells forming to eventually produce milk for her newborn. These "foreign cells" become the suspected culprits, the weakness between health and cancer.

In Chapter 10, I feared that my citing of the **Kevin Costner-Happy Family** article in McCall's Magazine, would be a jinx. I'm sad to report that he and his wife have filed for a divorce. It must be difficult to maintain balance and a sense of reality in glitzy Hollywood.

In March of 1996, Lorraine Mabbett (one of our Board members) and I attended the **First Conference for Directors of Crisis Pregnancy Centers** in Colorado Springs, Colorado. It was sponsored by Focus on the Family. There were over seven hundred and fifty of us attending, including a woman from Africa, who was trying to open a pregnancy clinic in her country. She sold some African art in order to get her return ticket home.

Dr. James Dobson, a Christian psychologist, the Director of Focus on the Family, has long been one of my heroes. I got to meet him. He's very tall, about 6 foot, 4 inches. He gave me a hug and congratulated me for having twenty-six years in the pro-life movement. He definitely is a "big man." He has been an unwavering champion of the unborn. His radio broadcasts and educational materials dealing with families are available worldwide.

In response to the **President's veto of HR 1833**, the partial-birth (D and X) abortion ban, Cardinals Joseph Bernardin, Anthony Bevilacqua, James Hickey, William Keeler, Bernard Law, Roger Mahony, Adam Maida, and John O'Connor sent an open letter to the President. Here is an excerpt from that letter:

# Update

> "It is with deep sorrow and dismay that we respond to your April 10 veto of the Partial-Birth Abortion Ban Act.
>
> "Your veto of this bill is beyond comprehension for those who hold human life sacred. It will ensure the continued use of the most heinous act to kill a tiny infant just seconds from taking his or her first breath outside the womb.
>
> "At the veto ceremony you told the American people that you "had no choice but to veto the bill." Mr. President, you and you alone had the choice of whether or not to allow children, almost completely born, to be killed brutally in partial-birth abortions...
>
> "During the veto ceremony you said you had asked Congress to change H.R. 1833 to allow partial-birth abortions to be done for "serious adverse health consequences" to the mother. You added that if Congress had included that exception, "everyone in the world will know what we're talking about.
>
> On the contrary, Mr. President, not everyone in the world would know that health, as the courts define it in the context of abortion, means virtually anything that has to do with a woman's overall "well-being...
>
> Writing this response to you in unison is, on our part, virtually unprecedented. It will, we hope, underscore our resolve to be unremitting and unambiguous in our defense of human life."

In my Epilogue I mentioned that I had not been able to meet **Norma McCorvey, (Jane Roe)** when I was in Dallas. That has since changed. I met her on June 14, 1996 at an Operation Rescue meeting in Southern California. She was a surprisingly good speaker. When I wrote about her initially I wondered if she had a low IQ. I noted that she appeared sleepy (possibly drugged?) when she made public appearances for the abortion advocates. In her speech on this particular night, she said she had been a drug-user and an alcoholic, but she has been drug- and alcohol-free since her conversion to Christianity. Her speech was intelligent and sincere. Before I went to the meeting, I had told my friends that I had mixed feelings about seeing Jane Roe—I really didn't admire her. Though I was glad she had changed her mind, I said that I couldn't applaud her. But, when I met her, after her talk, I did feel like hugging her. I welcomed her as a new Christian and as a new member of our pro-life family. Meeting her reminded me that all things are possible. I was renewed in my hope that my grandson and future grandchildren, might live in a country that regards all human life, including the unborn, as sacred and precious.

---

[1] Stephen Reinhardt, as quoted in *Los Angeles Times*, Times-Mirror Publising, March 7, 1996, page one, headline article.
Henry Weinstein, in "Assisted Deaths Ruled Legal," *Los Angeles Times*, March 7, 1996, p. 1.
Ibid.
*The Deadly After-Effect of Abortion: Breast Cancer*, Hayes Publishing Co., Inc., 6304 Hamilton Ave., Cincinnati, Ohio 45224.

# *Bibliography*

"**A Freedom Fighter Packs for Washington**" *Los Angeles Times* From, March 8, 1993, View section, p.1.

***A Private Choice***, John Noonan, The Free Press, McMillan Publishing, NY, 1979.

***Aborting America***, Bernard Nathanson, M.D., Doubleday & Company, Inc., Garden City, New York, 1979.

***Abortion & Social Justice***, Thomas W. Hilgers, in Hilgers and Horan, , Sheed & Ward, Inc., 1972.

***Abortion & the Christian***, John Jefferson Davis, Presbyterian and Reformed Publishing Co., Phillipsburg, NJ, 1984.

***Abortion and Social Justice***, Bart T. Heffernan, from a chapter, "The Early Biography of Every Man," in Sun Life, Thaxton, Virginia, 1980.

**Abortion and Women's Rights**, *ALL About Issues* magazine Frederica Mathewes-Green, published by American Life League, Virginia, March-April, 1992.

"**Abortion Bias Seeps Into News**," David Shaw, article in the *Los Angeles Times*, Times-Mirror Corp., July 1, 1990, p. 1.

***Abortion, Choice & Contemporary Fiction***, Judith Wilt, , University of Chicago Press, Chicago & London, 1990.

***Abortion: A Woman's Guide*** Alan Guttmacher, Planned Parenthood of New York City, Inc., Abelard-Schuman Ltd., 257 Park Ave., South, NewYork, NY, 10010, p. xii.

"**Abortion: Some Medical Facts**," National Right To Life Education Fund from the Pamphlet, entitled, published by the, 1984, 1988, 1989, 1991.

"**AIDS Knowledge, Perceived Risk and Prevention Among Adolescent Clients of a Family Planning Clinic**," C. S. Weisman, et al., *Family Planning Perspectives (FPP)*, Sep/Oct 1989.

***Anatomy of an Illness As Perceived by the Patient***, Cousins, Norman, , W. W. Norton & Company, Inc., New York, N.Y.., 173 pp.

***Backlash: The War Against American Women***, Susan Faludi Crown Publishers, Inc., NY, 1991.

***Bus 9 to Paradise***, Buscaglia, Leo, Fawcett-Columbine, NY, 1986.

"***Calif. Comm. on Therapeutic Abortion***," E. James Lieberman, "Informed Consent for Parenthood; Abortion and the Unwanted Children,", Springer, NY'71.

***Career Women and Childbearing*** Carole A. Wilk, , Van Nostrand Reinhold NY, 1986, p. 22.

"***Child and Family Reprint Booklet***," Herbert Ratner, M.D., "The Medical Hazards of the Birth Control Pill,", published by Child and Family Quarterly Magazine, Oak Park, Illinois, 1969.

"**Committee to Defend Reproductive Rights v. Myers**," 29 CAL. 3D 252 [1981].

"**Condoms for Kids? Get Real**," *Los Angeles Times*, Steven J. Sainsbury, M.D., July 13, 1993, Section B, p. 13.

***Daily News*, Los Angeles**, July 12, 1993, p. 10.

***Daily News,* Los Angeles**, June 17, 1993, front section, p. 3.

***Daily News,* Los Angeles**, Religion Section, "Los Angeles Catholic Census,", May 8, 1993.

# Bibliography

"**Dan Quayle Was Right**," *Atlantic Monthly*, Barbara Dafoe Whitehead, article in the, April 1993, p. 50.

**Doe v. Bolton**, 410 U.S., 179 [1973].

***Double Cross***, Denise Lardner Carmody, , Crossroad, NY, 1986, p. 119.

"**Examining the Roots of Judeo Christian Values**," Rabbi Daniel Lapin, from a radio broadcast of, Colorado Springs, Co., April, 1996.

***Fact Sheet***, "**Abortion and Waiting Period Requirements**," prepared by the Alan Guttmacher Institute for Planned Parenthood Federation of America, Inc. (FS-All, Rev. 1/93).

***Fact Sheet***, "**Teenage Women, Abortion, and the Law**," National Abortion Federation, August 1990.

***Family Planning Perspectives***, Alan Guttmacher Institute vol. 17, no. 2, March, April 1985, p. 85.

"**Fatherhood? Not Yet**," in, Focus on the Family, Colorado Springs, June 1993.

***For Every Idle Silence***, Henry Hyde, in, Servant Books, Ann Arbor, Michigan, 1985.

***Hollywood vs. America*** Michael Medved, , Harper Collins Publishers, NY, NY, 1992, p. 147.

***In the Clearing***, Frost, Robert, "Version," Holt, Rinehart and Winston, 1965, p. 37.

***Just the Facts*** brochure, published by Dayton Right to Life Society, 1990, Dayton, Ohio.

**Katz v. United States**, 389 U.S. 347,350 S. Ct.507 (1967).

***KKLA, FM Radio Broadcast***, Live from L.A., June 4, 1993, Jack Kocienski, the host.

***Life Advocate Magazine***, P. O. Box 13656, Portland, Oregon, 97213.

*Life Cycle* **pamphlet**, Jack Willke, M.D., from "When does Human Life Begin?" in, #108 (10/81), published by WCCL Education Fund, Inc., Milwaukee, Wis., 1981.

*Los Angeles Times,* Henry Weinstein, in "Assisted Deaths Ruled Legal,", March 7, 1996, p. 1.

*Los Angeles Times,* Leslie Berger, "Valley Case May Become test for 'Fetus Murder',", June 20, 1993, A 21.

*Los Angeles Times,* Stephen Reinhardt, as quoted in, Times-Mirror Publishing, March 7, 1996, page one, headline article.

*Margaret Sanger, an Autobiography* Sanger Margaret, , Maxwell Reprint Co., NY 1970, p. 55.

*Montel Williams Show*, KCOP-TV, Los Angeles, 3/17/93.

*Mother's Day is Over,* Shirley L. Radl, Charter House 1, NY 1973.

"**Nazism and Abortion**," *All About Issues* magazine, Don Feder, in e, March-April 1992, American Life League, Inc., Stafford Va., p. 14.

*One Generation After,* Elie Wiesel, , trans. by Lily Edelman and the author (New York: Random House, 1970.

*Orange County Register*, Friday, January 22, 1993, Section B1, p. 1.

**Planned Parenthood Los Angeles Information Sheet**, Public Affairs Department.

*Pregnancy and Childbearing* C. D. Hayes, ed., *Risking the Future: Adolescent Sexuality*, Vol. I, National Academy Press: Washington, D. C. 1987.

*Pro Life Answers to Pro Choice Arguments* Stanton, Elizabeth Cady, as cited by Randy

# Bibliography

Alcorn in, Multnomah Books, Questar Publishers, Sisters, Oregon, 1992.

**Rand Corporation's "Sex Survey,"** Santa Monica, Ca., May 1993.

*Report of the Commission on Population Growth and the American Future,* New American Library, New Am Library NY 1972.

**Right to Life Educational Foundation, Inc. Bulletin,** March, 1993, published by the Cincinnati Right to Life, Cincinnati, Ohio.

**Roe v. Wade,** 410 U. S. 113, 1973.

**"Sexual Harassment: Is There a Feminist Double Standard?"** *Ms. Magazine,* April 1993, p. 89.

*Single Issues,* Sobran, Joseph, The Human Life Press, NY, 1983, p. iv.

*Spiral Dance: A Rebirth of the Ancient Religion of the Great Goddess,* Starhawk, SF/Harper & Row, 1979.

**Supreme Court of the United States Syllabus,** Planned Parenthood of Southeastern Pennsylvania et al, v. Casey, Governor of Pennsylvania, et al., Daily Appellate Report, Tuesday, June 30, 1992.

**"The Abortions of Last Resort,"** Karen Tumulty, *Los Angeles Times Magazine,* 1/7/90, p. 10.

*The Center for Population Options,* August 1991.

**"The Church Search,"** Richard N. Ostling, *Time Magazine,* quoting Stephen D. Long, April 5, 1993, Time-Life Publishers.

*The Deadly After-Effect of Abortion: Breast Cancer,* Hayes Publishing Co., Inc., 6304 Hamilton Ave., Cincinnati, Ohio 45224.

*The Desolate City: Revolution in the Catholic Church,* Anne Roche Muggeridge, , Harper & Row, 1986.

*The Feminine Mystique* Friedan, Betty, , 20th Anniversary edition, W. W. Norton & Co., NY, 1983.

*The Gifts & Power of Woman*, Msgr. Paul J. Hayes, Daughters of St. Paul, Boston, 1987.

*The Index of Leading Cultural Indicators* William J. Bennett, , published jointly by Empower America, The Heritage Foundation, and Free Congress Foundation, Vol. I, March 1993, p. 15, and from U. S. Bureau of the Census, Current Population Reports, , p-20, No. 450, "Marital Status and Living Arrangements, 1991."

*The Missing Piece,* Ezell, Lee, , Servant Publications, Ann Arbor, Mich., 1992.

"**The New Activists: Fearless, Funny, Fighting Mad**," Louise Bernikow, in *Cosmopolitan Magazine*, April 1993, p. 162.

"**The Politics of Abortion**," *The Human Life Review*, Robert P. Casey, The Human Life Foundation, Inc., New York, N.Y. Summer 1992.

"*The Politics of Prayer, Feminist Language in the Worship of God*," Edited by Helen Hull Hitchcock, Ignatius Press, San Francisco, 1992.

*The Press and Abortion,* Marvin Olasky, Lawrence Erlbum Assoc., Hillsdale, NJ, 1988.

"**The Pro-life Principle Prevails: Dred Scott, Again**," Robert P. Casey, *Crisis, A Journal of Lay Catholic Opinion.*

*The Psychological Aspects of Abortion,* Sandra Mahkorn, "Pregnancy and Sexual Assault," Mall and Watts (1979).

*The Saturday Review,* Cousins, Norman, Oct. 16, 1971.

# Bibliography

*The Second Sex*, Simone De Bouvier, Alfred A. Knopf, NY 1952, p. 732.

*To Be A Woman in America*, Annette K.Baxter, , *1850-1930*, Times Books, NY 1978.

*Ungodly Rage*, Donna Steichen, , Ignatius Press, San Fracisco, 1991.

**Webster, Attorney General of Missouri v. Reproductive Health Services, et al.**, Court of Appeals, 8$^{th}$ Circuit, 88-605, [1989].

"Why are so Many Jews Liberal?" *Crisis Magazine, a Journal of Lay Catholic Opinion* Rabbi Daniel Lapin, in, , April, 1993.

"Why I No Longer Do Abortions," *Los Angeles Times*, George Flesh, M.D., 9/12/91, Op-Ed section.

"Why Is Everyone So Angry?," an interview of Dr. Dallas Willard of the University of Southern California, in *Focus on the Family Citizen Magazine* Colorado Springs, Co., Vol 7, No. 5, May 17, 1993, pp. 14 & 15.

*Why Johnny Can't Tell Right from Wrong* William K. Kilpatrick, , Simon & Schuster, NY, 1992.

*Women-church* Rosemary Ruether, , Harper & Row, San Francisco, 1985.

# Index

A to Z Women's Services, 190, 191
Addams, Jane, 183
Aid for Women, 192
AIDS, 107, 110, 119
Ainsworth, Mary, 102
Allred, Edward, 82
American Birth Control League, 26
American Civil Liberties Union, 48, 197
Assisted Suicides, 197

Baratta, Farnco, 28
Baxter, Annette, 183
Beezer, Judge Robert, 197
Bennett, William, 94
Bernardin, Cardinal Joseph, 162, 198
Bernikow, Louise, 131
Bevilacqua, Cardinal Anthony, 198
Black, Algernon, 27
Blackmun, Harry, 2, 15, 17, 23, 24, 37, 38
Bousha, Jill, 191
Boxer, Barbara, 40, 44, 193, 194
Breast Cancer, 198
Breedlove, Kirsten, 190, 191, 192
Brennan, William, 2
Brown, Helen Gurley, 87, 131
Burger, Warren, 2
Buscaglia, Leo, 1

Carmody, Denise Lardner, 140
Casey, Robert P., 14, 45, 46, 47, 53
Catholics for a Free Choice, 50, 142
Center for Populaton Options, 134
China, 197
Chlamydia, 109
Christian Coalition, 190, 192
Chung, Father Alex, 168

# Index

Cizmar, Reverend Tom, 169
Claremont Institute, 50
Clinica Feminina de l Comunidad, 79
Clinton, Bill & Hillary 1, 37, 38, 49, 198, 199
CNN, 129
Committee to Defend Reproductive Rights v. Myers, 7
Conrad, Paul, 129
Costner, Kevin, 133, 195, 198
Cousins, Norman, 2, 3
Coverdell, Senator, 194
Crisis Pregnancy Centers of Greater Phoenix, 18
Cummins, Mary, 34
Cusack, Father Thomas, 168

D and X Abortion, 9, 10, 64, 193, 194, 198, 199
Davis, Gray, 47
Davis, John Jefferson, 159
Dayton Right to Life Society, 147
de Bouvier, Simone, 182
Democratic National Convention, 46
Dilatation and Curettage, 65
Dilatation and Evacuation, 65
Dinkins, Mayor, 34
Distaval, 125
Dobson, Dr. James, 198
Doe v. Bolton, 5
Douglas, William, 2

Ectopic Pregnancy, 74
Edwards, Don, 44
Ehrlichman, John, 38
Elders, M. Joycelyn, 38, 39, 40, 196
Ethical Culture Society, 27
Euthanasia, 9, 193, 196
Eve Surgical Clinic, 58
Ezell, Lee, 77, 78

Faludi, Susan, 86, 178
Family Planning Associates, 81, 82, 150
Feder, Don, 30
Feinstein, Dianne, 44
Feminists for Life, 101
Fernandez, Joseph, 34
Finkbine, Sherri, 125, 126, 127, 130
Fisher, Bishop Carl, 168
Flesh, Dr. George, 59, 60, 72, 153
Focus on the Family, 31, 43, 198
Fogel, Julius, 87, 92
Foley, Thomas, 46
Foreman, Sherri, 28
Freedom of Choice Act, 44, 45
Friedan, Betty, iii,184, 185, 186
Frost, Robert, 1
Fuchs, Victor, 97

Geraldo, 108
Gieb, Eadie, 32
Gonorrhea, 110
Goodwin, Dr. Murphy, 194
Greene, A. C., 107
Guttmacher, Alan F., 74, 124
Guttmacher Institute, 110, 129

Haskell, Martin, 10, 56, 59, 64
Hatch, Senator Orrin, 53, 193
Hayes, Msgr. Paul J., 136, 137, 144, 163
Hayford, Pastor Jack, 169
Health, Education & Welfare, Dept. of, 38
Heffernan, Bart T., 57
Hellman, Louis, 38
Helms, Senator Jesse, 194
Her Medical Clnic, 47
Herpes, 109

# Index

Hickey, Cardinal James, 198
Hilgers, Dr. Thomas, 12
Hitchcock, Helen Hull, 138
Holocaust, The, 28
HR 1833, 198
Human papilomavirus, 109
Hunt, Mary, 50, 51, 52, 53, 142
Hyde, Representative Henry, 48, 53
Hyde Amendment, 43, 48
Hysterotomy, 66

Inhofe, Senator, 193, 194
Irving, Father Peter, 79, 168

Jackson, Jesse, 46
Jefferson, Thomas, 46
John Paul II, Pope, 168
Johnson, Magic, 107

Katz v. United States, 1
Keeler, Cardinal William, 198
Kennedy, Senator Ted, 194
Kennedy, Anthony, 14, 22, 24
Kilpatrick, William, 116, 117
Kindt, Esq., Anne J., 29
Kinneally, Leo, 64
KKLA-FM, 50
Kleegman, Sophia, 27
Koch, Ed, 49
Kocienski, Jack, 50
KROC Radio, 108, 113

Lader, Larry, 123, 159
Lapin, Rabbi Daniel, 31, 43, 170
Law, Cardinal Bernard, 198
Leibman, Abby J., 29

Levin, Michael, 137
Lieberman, E. James, 180
Lincoln, Abraham, 54
Littleton, Christine, 269
Living Will, 66
Long, Rev. D. Stephen, 170
Loop Center, 192

Mabbett, Lorraine, 198
Mahkorn, Dr. Sandra, 76
Mahony, Cardinal Roger, 198
Maida, Cardinal Adam, 198
Marks, Father Paul, 168
Marshall, Thurgood, 2
Mathewes-Green, Frederica, 101, 107, 176
Mc Mahan, James, 58, 64
McCarthy, Colmin, 87, 92
McCorvey, Norma 8, 127, 128, 130, 190, 199
Mecklenburg, Dr. Fred, 68
Medved, Michael, 98
Montrose, Colorado, 189
Muggeridge, Anne Roche, 123, 165

Nathanson, Dr. Bernard, 56, 57, 59, 123, 129, 159
National Abortion Federation, 10, 190
National Abortion Foundation, 130
National Abortion Rights Action League, 57
National Committee for a Human Life Amendment, 190, 192
National Committee on Maternal Health, 27, 124
National Organization of Women, 1, 184
National Right to Life Committee, 56
Natural Law, 50
Nixon, Richard, 37
Noonan, John, 53
Norplant, 36, 113, 114, 116, 119
Notre Dame Law School, 46

# Index

O'Connor, Cardinal John, 168, 196, 198
O'Connor, Sandra Day, 14, 22, 24
Olasky, Marvin, 27
Operation Rescue, 190
Ostling, Richard N. , 170

Packwood, Bob, 133
Pacoima, California, 47
Parents and Students United, 32
Partial Birth Abortions, 9, 10, 198
Personhood, 6,27, 30, 49
PlannedParenthood, 19, 39, 43, 45, 48, 82, 110, 111, 112, 115, 117, 124, 128, 149, 150, 152, 153, 154, 157, 164,
Powell, Lewis, 2
Privacy Right, 1, 6, 17, 28
Pro-Life Action League, 189, 192
Products of Conception, 149, 156, 157
Proposition 161, 21, 66, 67, 166
Prostaglandin Abortions, 65

Radl, Shirley L., 179
Rand Corporation, 33
Rape, 75, 77, 78
Ratner, Dr. Herbert, 112
Reagan, President Ronald, 5, 7
Rehnquist, Justice William, 2, 18, 22
Reinhardt, Stephen, 196, 197
Restell, Madame, 124
Reuther, Rosemary, 139, 140
Right to Life League of Southern California, ii, 29, 154, 169
Ripston, Ramona, 197
Robinson, Lamar, 190
Rockefeller III, John D., 38

Roe, Jane, 8, 199

Roe v. Wade, 1, 2, 4, 5, 8, 12, 20, 22, 24, 30, 34, 45, 46, 48, 49, 54, 130, 187
Roosevelt, Eleanor, 182
RU-486, i

Sainsbury, Dr. Steven J., 115
Saint Paul, 143, 144
Salt Poisoning, 65
San Fernando High School, 113
Sanchez, Angela, 79
Sanger, Margaret, 26, 37
Scalia, Justice Antonin, 18, 20, 22, 23
Scheidler, Joseph, 189, 192
Scott, Dred, 23, 30, 31, 46, 54, 67
Shaw, David, 128
Shields, Brooke, 107
*Shirley Valentine,* 178, 179
Smith, Congressman Chris, 53
Smith, Senator Robert, 193
Sochen, June, 182
Souter, David, 14, 24
Spalding, Matt, 50
Stanton, Elizabeth Cady, 26
Starhawk, 140
Steichen, Donna, 138
Stevens, Mary, 189
Steward, Potter, 2
Suction Aspiration, 64
Syphilis, 106, 109, 110

Teresa, Mother, 168
Thalidomide, 125
*Thelma and Louise,* 178
Therapeutic Abortion Act, 7
Thomas, Justice Clarence, 18, 20, 22

*Toward Tradition*, 170
Tumulty, Karen, 58

Vaughn, Bishop Austin, 168
Ver Burg, Pastor Bob, 169
Viability, 5, 8

Webster v. Reproductive Health Services, 6,
Weisel, Elie, 59
White, Justice Byron White, 2, 18, 22
Whitehead, Barbara Dafoe, 96, 97, 98, 103
Wilk, Carole A., 86, 99, 101, 102
Williams, Montel, 108
Willke, Dr. Jack, 56
Wilt, Judith, 141
Women-church, 139, 140
Women's Alliance for Theology, Ethics and Ritual, 50
Women's Center, 192
Women's Law Center, 29
Wyden, Ron, 130

*Gail Hamilton* has spoken with and counseled thousands of women in the last twenty-six years. She is a past Board Member of the Right to Life League of Southern California, and continues as the Director of the Pregnancy Counseling Clinic in Mission Hills, California. She frequently speaks to adults and students of all ages.

She lives with her husband, Michael, and their sixteen-year-old daughter, Susan, in the San Fernando Valley. They have two older daughters, one son, and one grandson.

A percentage of all profits from this book will be donated to the Pregnancy Counseling Clinic of Mission Hills, California, a tax-deductible, non-profit organization.

You may write Mrs. Hamilton in care of Family of Man Publishing, P. O. Box 17328, Encino, Ca. 91416-17328.